Work and Men

An Employers' Guide

Edited by Doreen M. Miller, Maurice Lipsedge
and Paul Litchfield

Gaskell & Faculty of Occupational Medicine

© The Royal College of Psychiatrists 2002
Cover artwork © Ian Whadcock 2002/eastwing.co.uk

Gaskell is an imprint of the Royal College of Psychiatrists, 17 Belgrave Square, London SW1X 8PG
http://www.rcpsych.ac.uk

British Library Cataloguing-in-Publication Data.
A catalogue record for this book is available from the British Library.
ISBN 1-901242-85-4

Distributed in North America by Balogh International Inc.

The views presented in this book do not necessarily reflect those of the Royal College
of Psychiatrists, and the publishers are not responsible for any error of omission or fact.

The Royal College of Psychiatrists is a registered charity (no. 228636).
Printed by Bell & Bain Limited, Glasgow, UK.

This publication is sponsored Swiss Life (UK) plc

Swiss Life (UK) plc provide life, critical illness and income protection
products to employees and individuals, offering financial security during
times of need: death, disability and illness. We are one of the UK's largest
employee benefits protection providers, covering more than 1.6 million
employees and their families, in approximately 8000 group schemes.

More specifically, we are also one of the UK's largest providers of group
income protection, providing an income to employees during ill health.
And as such, we are all too aware of the growth in mental health problems
and illness. We aim to work with employers and individuals wherever
possible to set in place measures:

- to prevent mental illness in the first place.
- to rehabilitate and encourage those who have had to take time off
  work due to mental illness, back to work.

We are delighted therefore to sponsor *Work and Mental Health: An Employers'
Guide*, which aims to promote good practice in the field of mental health at
work. We hope that the inclusion of practical programmes that deal with
mental health workplace issues proves a valuable resource to employers
and human resources professionals.

Graham Clark
Director, Employee Benefits, Swiss Life (UK) plc

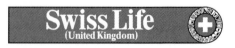

Contents

List of tables, boxes and figures   v

List of contributors   vii

Preface   x

Introduction   xi
Paul Litchfield

Acknowledgement   xiii

1   Management of change: the Glaxo Pharmaceuticals case study   1
    Bill Proudlock

2   Legal aspects of mental health in the workplace   10
    Denis D'Auria, Gillian Howard and Peter Verow

3   Risk management approach to mental health: the London
    Electricity case study   23
    Anne Margaret Samuel

4   Mental well-being in the workplace: building the business case   28
    Noeleen Doherty

5   Developing a mental health policy: an outline   34
    Ann Fingret

6   Individual and organisational stress   47
    Marian Roden and Stephen Williams

7   A team approach to managing mental health at work:
    the AstraZeneca case study   53
    Richard Heron

8   Managing pressure: the Marks & Spencer case study   60
    Noel McElearney

9 Supporting mental well-being through the promotion of a balanced lifestyle 68
Marian Roden

10 Assessing mental health problems in the workplace 75
Matthew Hotopf and Janet Carruthers

11 Anxiety, depression, suicide risk, bullying and occupational health interventions 82
Maurice Lipsedge and Anne Margaret Samuel

12 Substance misuse/addiction: alcohol 98
Paul Gwinner and David Moore

13 Substance misuse/addiction: drugs 105
C. C. H. Cook and Graham Bell

14 Anorexia and bulimia 109
J. H. Lacey and N. A. Mitchell-Heggs

15 The effects of travel on mental well-being: fear of flying and other psychiatric disorders 114
Su Wang and Lawrence Burns

16 Critical incidents and violence at work 121
Ian Palmer and Charles Baron

17 Chronic fatigue syndrome 127
Michael Sharpe and Derek White

18 Schizophrenia and delusional disorders 132
Trevor Turner and Paul Litchfield

19 Organic states 138
Chris Ball and Alan Scott

20 Personality disorders in the workplace 144
Alison Martin, Maurice Lipsedge and James Watson

21 The role of mental health professionals 148
Steve McKeown and Susan Robson

22 The role of the liaison psychiatrist 154
Andrew Hodgkiss and David Snashall

Index 159

Tables, boxes and figures

Tables

5.1 Landmarks of the developing interest in occupational
    mental health   35

5.2 The four organisational styles and their effects on
    employee well-being   39

5.3 Changes and procedures to improve the person–
    environment fit   44

6.1 The most common and important workplace stressors   48

8.1 The PMI sub-scales   63

10.1 Occupational toxins and psychiatric disorders   77

11.1 Comparison of anxiety disorders in terms of duration and
    specificity to certain situations   86

12.1 Individual factors   99

15.1 Annual medical in-flight incidents recorded by one
    international airline   115

15.2 Estimates of how long jet lag will last   118

17.1 A hypothetical causal model of CFS   128

18.1 The key symptoms of schizophrenia   133

19.1 Organic *v.* functional psychiatric problems   141

Boxes

2.1 The Farnsworth case   10

2.2 The O'Brien case   11

2.3 The leading case for unfair dismissal on the grounds
    of ill health   19

2.4 The Kapadia case   21

4.1 The cost of mental ill health to business   29

4.2 The Walker case: setting a precedent   30

4.3 Barclays Bank   31

4.4 Consignia   32

10.1 Preliminaries for the interview   76

10.2 The psychiatric history   76

10.3 The Mental State Examination 79
10.4 Asking questions about suicide 80
10.5 Key questions in diagnosis 80
10.6 Types of problems appropriate for referral 81
11.1 The differential diagnosis of generalised anxiety and
     panic disorder 85
11.2 Symptoms common to both anxiety and depression 89
12.1 Policy on alcohol 103
14.1 The five SCOFF questions 112
14.2 Relevant information to seek in potential cases of
     eating disorder 113
15.1 Factors which may affect a traveller's coping capacity 119
17.1 Core aspects of case definition of chronic fatigue syndrome 127
17.2 Summary of the treatment approaches for CFS 130

Figures

3.1 The costs of managing mental health 24
3.2 Model of risk assessment used in London Electricity's
    Fit For Work programme 24
3.3 Functional mismatch: the balance between work demands
    and the worker's capability 26
3.4 Comparison of outcomes on the motivation RIAT measure 26
3.5 Comparison of outcomes on the work demands RIAT measure 27
6.1 The relationship between pressure, growth and stress 48
7.1 Reasons for staff consulting the CALM team 56
8.1 The dynamics of the stress process 62
8.2 Different sources of pressure combine to interact with
    personality and experience 64
9.1 The relationship between pressure and performance,
    and its dependence upon individual resilience 72
9.2 The three prerequisites of organisational capability 73
11.1 The cognitive model of acute anxiety 84
12.1 A simple model of the presentation of alcohol problems
     in an employee 101

Contributors

Chris Ball MRCPsych, Consultant and Senior Lecturer in Old Age Psychiatry, South London and Maudsley NHS Trust, Ladywell Unit, Lewisham High Street, Lewisham, London SE13 6LH

Charles Baron FFOM FRCP, Consultant Occupational Physician, Flintshire County Council

Graham Bell MB ChB MSc FFOM DA DIH, Occupational Health Department, Esso Petroleum Co. Ltd, Mailpoint 04, Ermyn Way, Leatherhead KT22 8UX

Lawrence Burns BSc DAP(Clin.) PhD ABPsS FRSH, Consultant Clinical Psychologist, The Altincham Priory Hospital, Hale, Cheshire

Janet Carruthers FFOM MSc, Consultant Occupational Physician, Department of Occupational Health and Safety, King's College Hospital, Denmark Hill, London SE5 9RS

C.C.H. Cook MD MRCPsych, Professor of the Psychiatry of Alcohol Misuse, Consultant Psychiatrist, Kent Institute of Medicine and Health Sciences, University of Kent at Canterbury, Canterbury, Kent CT2 7PD

Denis D'Auria MA LLM MD DIH DipMedEd DipRCPath FFOM, Consultant Occupational Physician and Director, Legge Hunter Centre, Barts and The London NHS Trust, St Bartholomew's Hospital, West Smithfield, London EC1A 7BE, and Honorary Senior Lecturer, St Bartholomew's and Royal London School of Medicine and Dentistry, Queen Mary University, London

Noeleen Doherty PhD Visiting Fellow, Cranfield School of Management, Cranfield University, Cranfield, Bedford MK43 0AL

Ann Fingret MB BS FFOM FFOM (RCPI), Consultant Occupational Physician, c/o The Royal College of Psychiatrists, 17 Belgrave Square, London SW1X 8PG

Paul Gwinner MRCPsych DPM AFOM, Consultant Psychiatrist, Prena UK, Redditch, Worcestershire B98 0DU

Richard Heron FRCP FFOM, Head of Global Safety, Health and Risk Management and Principal Medical Officer, AstraZeneca, Alderley House, Alderley Park, Macclesfield, Cheshire SK10 4TF

Andrew Hodgkiss MD MRCPsych, Consultant Liaison Psychiatrist, South London and Maudsley NHS Trust and St Thomas' Hospital; Honorary Senior Lecturer in Liaison Psychiatry, Guy's, King's and St Thomas' School of Medicine, St Thomas' Hospital, London SE1 7EH

Matthew Hotopf PhD MRCPsych, Reader in Psycholgical Medicine, Department of Psychological Medicine, Institute of Psychiatry, 103 Denmark Hill, London SE5 8AZ

Gillian Howard LLB DipCompLaw (Cantab) Hon FFOM, Employment Lawyer and Consultant to Gordon Dadds, Mayfair Solicitors, 34 Lyndale Avenue, London NW2 2QA

J. H. Lacey MD MPhil FRCPsych, Professor of Psychiatry, St George's Hospital Medical School, Cranmer Terrace, London SW17 0RE

Maurice Lipsedge MPhil FRCP FRCPsych FFOM(Hon), Emeritus Consultant Psychiatrist, The South London and Maudsley NHS Trust, Honorary Senior Lecturer in the Department of Psychological Medicine, Guy's, King's and St Thomas' School of Medicine, Head of Section of Occupational Psychiatry and Psychology, Keats House, 24–26 St Thomas Street, London SE1 9RS

Paul Litchfield OStJ MSc FRCP FFOM, Chief Medical Officer and Head of Health and Safety, BT Group plc, 81 Newgate Street, London EC1A 7AJ

Alison Martin MFOM MIOSH, Regional Medical Director, BP International Ltd

Noel McElearney MSc FFOM FFOM(I), Director, Group Medical Services, Scottish and Newcastle plc, 33 Ellersly Road, Edinburgh EH12 6HX

Steve McKeown MB BS MRCPsych FFOM, Consultant Psychiatrist, Medical Director, Cheadle Royal Health Care Services, Cheadle Royal Hospital, 100 Wilmslow Road, Cheadle, Cheshire SK8 3DG

N. A. Mitchell-Heggs FRCP FFOM DCH, Consultant Occupational Physician, St George's Hospital and Medical School, London

David Moore MB BS DPH DTM&H DIH FFOM, formerly Director of Group Medical Services, Scottish and Newcastle plc, Holyrood Road, Edinburgh EH8 8YS (retired)

Ian Palmer MRCPsych, Tri-Service Professor of Defence Psychiatry, Royal Centre for Defence Medicine, K Block, Sellyoak Hospital, Raddlebarn Road, Sellyoak, Birmingham B29 6JD

Bill Proudlock PhD FCIPD Former Human Resources Director, Glaxo Wellcome UK, and current Chair, Pharmaceuticals Industry National Training Organisation, c/o The Royal College of Psychiatrists, 17 Belgrave Square, London SW1X 8PG

Susan Robson FFOM FRCP, County Medical Health and Safety Adviser, Cheshire County Council

Marian Roden MA MB BS AFOM, formerly Senior Medical Director, SmithKline Beecham Pharmaceuticals, The Frythe, Welwyn, Hertfordshire AL6 9AR

Anne Margaret Samuel MSc FRCP FFOM, Group Occupational Physician, Occupational Health Department, London Electricity, 34–38 Aybrook Street, London W1M 3JL

Alan Scott FFOM, Senior Medical Inspector, Health and Safety Executive, Honorary Staff Physician in Accident and Emergency Medicine, University Hospital, Nottingham

Michael Sharpe MA MD MRCP MRCPsych, Reader in Psychological Medicine, University of Edinburgh, Kennedy Tower, Royal Edinburgh Hospital, Edinburgh EH10 5HF

David Snashall MSc FRCP FFOM LLM, Senior Lecturer in Occupational Medicine, Guy's, King's and St Thomas' School of Medicine, Head of Service, Occupational Health Department, Guy's and St Thomas' Hospital Trust; Chief Medical Adviser, Health and Safety Executive

Trevor Turner MD FRCPsych, Consultant Psychiatrist and Clinical Director, East London and The City Mental Health NHS Trust, Homerton Hospital, Homerton Row, London E9 6SR

Peter Verow MB BS FFOM, Occupational Health Unit, Sandwell Health Care, 30 Hallam Close, Hallam Street, West Bromwich B91 4HU

Su Wang MFOM MSc DIH DPH, Consultant Occupational Physician, The Post Office, 148 Old Street, London EC1V 9HQ

James Watson MD FRCP FRCPsych, The Guy's, King's College and St Thomas' Hospitals' Medical and Dental School, Division of Psychiatry and Psychology, Guy's Hospital, London

Derek White MRCGP FRCP FFOM, Chief Medical Officer, British Telecommunications plc, 81 Newgate Street, London EC1A 7AJ

Stephen Williams PhD, Organisational Psychologist, Managing Director, Resource Systems, Claro Court, Claro Road, Harrogate HG1 4BA

Preface

It is a pleasure for us to have been invited to write this preface as this book represents a significant meeting of minds and the application of the unique skills of our respective disciplines to the issues of mental health in the workplace. The Presidents of the Royal College of Psychiatrists and the Faculty of Occupational Medicine, even within the academy of medical Royal Colleges, would not normally be perceived to have much in common in the practice of their respective specialities, but this book shows how wrong such a perception is. It is apt that the workplace should be the common denominator.

The outcomes of two major initiatives to broaden understanding of the issues of mental health and work have been brought together to produce a superb source of practical material, of equal value to the psychiatrist and occupational physician. These were a joint meeting of the Faculty and Society of Occupational Medicine on 'Mental Well-being in the Workplace – Current Practice' and 'The ABC of Mental Health for Occupational Physicians', a series of concise leaflets distributed with the Faculty's newsletter. The specialist knowledge of the authors, who are occupational physicians, psychiatrists and chartered clinical psychologists, is harnessed synergistically, making the value and authority of each section greater than the sum of its parts.

The topics covered are current, reflecting today's problems in the context of working in Britain in the 21st century. The prevention of mental ill health in the workplace is as important as managing it, for sound social and economic reasons. This book will play a major role in destigmatising mental illness in the workplace and will demonstrate that mental illness is no bar to working effectively – a process in itself beneficial.

Perhaps most important of all, the hard work that each author and the editors have put into this book demonstrates a fundamental tenet of medical practice – doctors and other health care professionals working together in the best interests of their patients.

John Cox
President, Royal College of Psychiatrists
Jim Sykes
President, Faculty of Occupational Medicine

Introduction

Paul Litchfield

The focus of concern in relation to health at work has shifted in recent years from physical illness and injury to mental health. The post-industrial economies of the Western world expose far fewer employees, at least in their own countries, to physical hazards and where such hazards remain they are generally well controlled, by historical standards. However, the pace and the intensity of work in our society has increased substantially as multinational corporations compete in the global marketplace and this has brought with it previously unimagined pressures on those in employment. These pressures are occurring at a time of unprecedented change in both the business world and society. The old certainties of job security, at least for those in white-collar employment, and hierarchical structures have been replaced by more dynamic and fluid organisations and conditions of employment. In parallel the traditional family structure, with its inherent support mechanisms, is becoming the exception as more women enter employment and lifelong marriage is no longer the norm. 'Stress' has become common parlance in both the boardroom and on the shop floor and, perhaps predictably, a whole industry offering solutions, of varying efficacy, from aromatherapy to zen has developed.

Despite the media hyperbole and the pseudo-science that tends to surround stress at work, there is no doubt that mental health is an issue of real importance to employers and employees alike. The Health and Safety Executive estimates that 6.5 million working days were lost in Britain in 1995 due to stress, depression, anxiety or a physical condition ascribed to work stress. This equates to a direct cost to employers of some £370 million and the estimated cost to society as a whole is £3.75 billion. Mental illness now vies with musculoskeletal disorders as the commonest cause of sickness absence and ill health retirement in many companies. Litigation for personal injury resulting from psychosocial hazards is becoming increasingly common and expensive, while the authorities are directing substantial effort into encouraging employers to adopt a risk management approach in this area. These potential costs to business are important, but enlightened employers are looking beyond these loss control and compliance aspects to enhancing performance through the promotion of mental well-being.

This book brings together the series of articles published by the Faculty of Occupational Medicine – 'The ABC of Mental Health for Occupational Physicians' – as well as presentations from a conference organised by the Society of Occupational Medicine, entitled 'Mental Well-being in the Workplace – Current Practice'. Both elements aim to describe good practice in the field of mental health at work and give practical descriptions of programmes implemented by some of the leading companies operating in the UK. This is a fast-evolving area of practice and each organisation will need to develop programmes which suit its own culture and business needs. However, it is hoped that the material contained in this book will provide a stimulus to develop such programmes and be a source of ideas which can be adapted and refined.

Acknowledgement

Our thanks to Ramona Nock, Project Coordinator at Miller Health Management, for her invaluable contribution to the publication of this book.

CHAPTER 1

Management of change:
the Glaxo Pharmaceuticals case study

Bill Proudlock

Introduction

Most employees would argue that the best thing management could do for their mental well-being would be to slow the pace of change. Modern businesses are preoccupied with the need to change because they are operating in increasingly complex and dynamic, if not unstable, marketplaces. The globalisation of markets, the search for economies of scale, the compression of technological advance and the commoditisation of products are a few of the typical pressures on businesses. Even if a business tried to ignore them, the stock market or pressure from a regulator would soon bring it to heel.

Practitioners in change management often observe that companies develop elegant strategies for change – usually beautifully documented to impress the City or the regulators. One leading academic has remarked that such wonderful strategies are unlikely to produce a competitive advantage as their competitors have probably used the very same consultants to devise a similar strategy!

What is more rarely observed is a coherent programme for implementing a business strategy: in particular, a plan which outlines how the organisation proposes to alter people's behaviours, attitudes and working practices so that they can operate effectively in these new and ever more complex environments. All too often this most critical part of the change process is expected to happen automatically after senior management has identified a pressing need for change. Translating the vision into practice typically involves a video message from senior management, some change management workshops and a T-shirt if communication is seen as important! It is therefore unsurprising that change programmes have a bad name for upsetting the mental well-being of employees.

If change came in controlled modules and in an orderly sequence, employees and organisational cultures might adapt spontaneously, without planned support for implementation. In practice, as the following case study shows, changes in business rarely come singly or in a neat order. Glaxo Pharmaceuticals UK (GPUK) had planned a powerful support programme for a major re-engineering in 1994 but what could not have been anticipated was that the change would coincide with a merger with Wellcome UK.

The changing nature of the workforce

Any change in life can be stressful, but overload commonly arises when there is a confluence of changes or other pressures. Many businesses experienced major organisational change during the 1970s and the 1980s but it could be argued that, for most employees, family or private life was generally relatively stable. However, this was not the case during the 1990s. Changes in society removed traditional support mechanisms for many and patterns of social relationship became infinitely more complex for most. In consequence, pressures at work were likely to be matched by pressures at home, with a higher risk of impairment of employees' mental well-being.

The increasing dependence of organisations on 'knowledge workers' has also affected the way in which organisations have to approach the management of change. Companies such as GPUK began to recognise in the late 1980s that their future success would be in the hands of 'Generation X' people. This group had radically different expectations of work and life to those of their predecessors, and they were also the generation experiencing, at first hand, the changes in the social fabric. These people, who would be in the engine room of change for the company, were the group whose mental well-being was most likely to be affected by poorly implemented programmes and the least likely to suffer in silence.

These drivers increasingly led companies to realise that no business strategy can be regarded as complete without a support programme to help ensure that changes are implemented with the minimum disruption to employees' mental well-being. The consequences of not doing so – as a senior manager involved in a recent merger between two companies with rather traditional attitudes learned – are significant. He noted that 'they give us a new organisation chart today and expect us to operate it effectively tomorrow!' It was therefore not surprising that morale in his unit was low, stress levels were high and energy for the post-merger tasks limited.

By providing its employees with support, an organisation not only demonstrates that it values them but it also increases the likelihood that it will successfully implement the desired strategy. Since many companies are in a process of continuous change and adaptation, it is important for them to recognise that quick fixes will not help them meet their objectives and that long-term support programmes are required. However, the costs of properly constructed support programmes are significant and are rarely considered in the initial costing of business change. Exposing these costs can alter the economics of a change, such as a merger, and can encourage questions concerning the time it will take to achieve the planned benefits. Reality is often an unwelcome guest when promises of speedy benefits have been made to senior management, the City or a regulator.

All this places an enormous responsibility on the leadership of companies facing business change. More particularly, it brings into stark relief the role of practitioners in human resources (HR) and occupational health and their real influence on the business. It is their job to ensure that structured programmes to support implementation are developed, that costs are calculated and that the programme is implemented as an integral part of the overall business change. The experience of GPUK in managing the massive changes which affected their market in the late 1980s and then into the 1990s can be used to illustrate these points.

GPUK: a case study

The first stage in helping employees to deal effectively with change is for companies to predict events and to assess their likely effect on staff. At GPUK, in the late 1980s, the organisation's scenario-based planning process brought to light the significant impact changes within the National Health Service (NHS), which was GPUK's principal customer, would have on the whole organisation. At the time, the organisation predicted that the forthcoming five years would be 'turbulent'. In retrospect, this prediction was a gross understatement.

During this period, the plans that were put forward to help the organisation adapt to the identified changes suggested that, 'to be as successful in the 1990s as we had been in the 1980s, we would have to make huge changes in our attitudes, behaviours and working practices'. In essence, the organisation had to bring about a change in culture to match the changes in the marketplace. At the same time, the company also faced a relocation, several major product launches and changes in regulation. It soon became apparent that the organisation could not continue to operate as it had done previously and that, because of the sheer magnitude of change, the mental well-being of employees could be affected.

Employees' attitudes to change

Surveys carried out at this time revealed that employees were anxious about the impending changes. Although they felt confident that the powerful Glaxo management team would continue to be successful, they did not believe that management had the power to influence the impact that these changes would have on their own personal situations. Essentially, they did not really trust management to look after them.

The employee survey also showed a rigid, functionally based structure with a pace of decision-making that matched that style. This was unsurprising, as the company had been hugely successful in the 1980s, was twice the size of its nearest competitor and enjoyed established relationships with its key contacts in the NHS. To use a military analogy redolent of the period, it was structured like the forces of NATO at the height of the Cold War, well prepared to meet the Russian tank armies on the North German plain but ill equipped for guerrilla warfare. The board of the company recognised these challenges and decided that success could be maintained only through a programme of behavioural change to prepare staff for the trials to come. At the time this was not seen in the specific context of caring for the mental well-being of employees but rather as a critical component in securing the future of the business. In retrospect, failure to adopt such a support programme would have compromised the success of the company and could have seriously damaged the mental well-being of employees.

Changing the organisational culture

The culture change programme which was introduced was called Developing for the '90s. Within this programme the behavioural precepts considered necessary for future success were identified as:

(1)   role clarity
(2)   acceptance of change
(3)   teamwork
(4)   innovation
(5)   output orientation.

The initial phase of the programme consisted of asking the top 200 managers to assess whether they considered these the right precepts to ensure success against the demands of the scenario. Broad and enthusiastic agreement was obtained – one usefully reordered the precepts to provide the acronym RATIO.

Once the senior managers had understood the magnitude of the changes and the impact on their staff, they took some positive steps to secure their own mental well-being. They said to the board: 'We think this is a great approach and we think you're serious – but this will work only if *all* employees go through the programme'. Originally the intention had been to limit training to senior managers, who would in turn cascade this information down to their staff. Faced with this demand, Sean Lance, the Managing Director and later Chief Operating

Officer of Glaxo Wellcome plc, took an instant and instinctive decision to extend the programme. This was not an easy decision because there was no money in the budget and the initial programme had been seen as too adventurous by some powerful senior figures. Furthermore, if the programme had not shown early success, the credibility of the Managing Director and the Human Resources Director would have been irreparably damaged. Fortunately, shortly afterwards, GPUK secured the Chairman's Award as the highest-performing unit in Glaxo. A number of other companies in the UK, such as Unilever, BP and Hewlett Packard, announced similar responses to change at that time but none appeared to support them with the level of resource applied by GPUK.

During this period the relocation to a new site had allowed a different approach to be taken to the provision for occupational health. This consisted of a system based on occupational health advisers who reported to the human resources function; strong professional support and standard setting were supplied by an occupational physician. Although the change was not effected without tensions, a real partnership began to develop between the human resources and occupational health teams. This meant that issues of mental well-being were more explicitly addressed when the change strategies were reviewed. Partnership meant both a more sophisticated approach to the management of mental health issues in the workplace and, more importantly, an increasingly effective input into the issues raised with occupational health by employees consulting them during times of change. This helped to keep human resources policy makers in touch with the practical impact of change implementation.

At the same time as the structure of the company was changing, so was its composition. GPUK had recently expanded to some 1500 employees, 700 of whom were in field-selling and support. This expansion had led to a significant increase in the number of women employed in professional and managerial roles: increases of approximately 50% in selling and 35% in management. While it is not possible to quantify the effect of gender on the culture change programme, it was widely believed that women exerted a significant influence in gaining acceptance for the new, more open and less competitive ways of working.

By the early 1990s it was believed the culture had moved from the Cold War, heavy-armour style described earlier to that of a crack light infantry regiment. However, even this was not enough to fully equip it for the guerrilla warfare of the developing marketplace and it was felt that the organisation would have to move to an even more flexible/ organic style – perhaps more SAS than conventional infantry! The accepted view was that if the organisation could learn to mould and adapt itself to changing scenarios it would be more effective as well as being a fun place to work. This was important because throughout this period of massive reorganisation the culture change programme fostered the idea that, while employees were expected to be passionate about business success, they were also expected to have fun, and that this would have beneficial effects on mental well-being.

The model for mental well-being that was now emerging was no longer purely reactive, relying on the existence of support systems for those whose mental health had broken down and stress management courses to help employees cope when things were going wrong. Rather, it was based on the quality of the strategic planning process, its ability to anticipate the impact of change on employees, and management's success in providing the methodologies to change behaviours so that they were suited to the needs of the new marketplace. This is in no way to denigrate or deny the need for these other mechanisms, but they can only cure and repair, not prevent.

It is not possible to say with absolute certainty that instituting a process of culture change helped to maintain the mental well-being of GPUK's employees through the early 1990s but successive employment surveys over that period suggested a strong positive effect on morale. Conviction increased that reorganisation had to be backed up by support programmes to help employees understand, accept and be involved in the process of change.

Reorganisation

As predicted, change did not stop after the initial changes were effected in the NHS. Interfaces with the NHS became more complex, particularly for those in field-sales, and further significant changes in organisation and working practices appeared necessary as the market seemed to become less stable. In 1994, GPUK decided it needed to reorganise along process lines and began working with Boston Consulting to establish the appropriate organisational style and structure for the end of the decade and beyond. The new initiative was not cheap, in terms of either fees or the effort required to keep the business running during the change process. There was a great temptation to allow the implementation to proceed without further support programmes of the RATIO type, with all of the associated risk and expense. However, the temptation was resisted because it was recognised that most employees would need to change jobs, present themselves against new roles with new competencies and manage two roles during the transition. The potential impact on mental well-being was enormous and it was recognised that it could jeopardise effective implementation.

People do not react well to changes when preoccupied with the thought that 'I'm having to reapply for my job'. While senior management and the consultants may have seen the 'new job' as a vibrant, exciting new opportunity, a worried employee with a big mortgage and a partner facing change in another organisation may have had a different perspective. It was recognised that, while the organisation could not allay all of an employee's anxieties, it could help alleviate some of concerns if the principles of procedural justice (Kim & Mauborgue, 1997) were adopted. The aim was to ensure that procedures for allocating people to new roles not only were fair but also were perceived to be fair.

Two major responses emerged to support employees affected by the implementation of this new organisation and style. The first was the appointment of behavioural change consultants and the second was the provision of occupational health support. Two teams of adventurous behavioural change consultants, Alexander and Bridge, were appointed to support the key management teams who had to implement the changes. Both consultancies were at the forefront of behavioural and leadership development, were very ready to challenge established practices and provided tailor-made support to both groups and individuals. This proved to be very successful, as shown by the positive reaction of employees in a survey that was conducted by the Leading Edge Forum Ltd, led by Professor Lynda Gratton of London Business School (Gratton, 1997). However, the most significant outcome of the intervention was that GPUK employees developed exceptionally strong competencies in change management.

The second response arose out of discussions between the human resources and occupational health departments about the impact the pace of change was having on the organisation and its employees. Consideration was given to the provision of an employee helpline, which had proved successful in other contexts, but this was not seen as a sufficiently powerful response to the radical changes in the GPUK reorganisation. Employees' difficulties almost always revolved around mental well-being and it was thought that they could best be supported by channelling their concerns through the occupational health department. Initially, the department offered employees professional counselling as needed, through an external group, Kensington Counselling. However, in view of the strong partnership that had developed between the occupational health and human resources departments, and increasingly line managers, this rapidly developed into a well-publicised and well-understood support service for both employees and managers. In retrospect, its open existence seemed to enhance the ability of employees and managers to deal effectively and more openly with issues of mental well-being.

During the extended period of implementation, both processes served GPUK extremely well. Managers implementing complex changes felt supported by their work with Alexander and Bridge, both as individuals and in their teams. Both consultancies operated with individuals and teams on a confidential basis (there was no feedback without consent). In addition, when problems arose around the mental well-being of any of their team members, there was a clearly defined and well publicised route to professional counselling, which could be initiated by the individual or their manager, using well-structured guidelines.

Early on in the reorganisation it became apparent that a large proportion of the employees using the occupational health department/Kensington system had a dominant issue outside the work environment. It was found that the major external issue affecting employees was a relationship problem and for many the changes in the workplace were the 'final straw' in an already overloaded emotional life. With hindsight this was not surprising since most of the employees affected were in their twenties or thirties and under peak career and personal pressures. The initial assumption had been the simplistic one that it was the reorganisation which would be the principal problem and, indeed, work change was usually the reason the employee first gave when attending the occupational health department. These findings amply demonstrate how the increasingly complex interactions between business and personal lives and relationships significantly affect mental well-being in the workplace.

Midway through this complex and challenging implementation, GPUK merged with another large pharmaceutical company, Wellcome UK. This resulted in another wave of significant change, involving new products and the assimilation of a large tranche of additional employees into a newly developed culture. Further, the change programme began to overlap with issues concerning the loss of patent protection on Glaxo's major product, Zantac (ranitidine, a medication for ulcers). As this phase progressed, the pattern of referrals to the occupational health department/Kensington changed and became more dominated by sheer pressure of business change, although often exacerbated by domestic or personal issues. This was an interesting reversal from the earlier pattern and perhaps reflects the cumulative effect of serial change.

Conclusion

The period described was one of dramatic business turbulence and there is no doubt that there were some employees who suffered upset or harm as a result. However, the model adopted by GPUK provides an example of how occupational health and human resources professionals can provide directed and effective programmes to minimise the impact of change on the mental well-being of employees.

The key success factors for any organisation seeking to manage change effectively are:

(1)   a meaningful vision of its future operating scenarios
(2)   an ability to forecast the new behaviours and working practices needed to function effectively in those scenarios

(3)   the will to commit the necessary time, effort and money to powerful support programmes.

It may be easier to persuade senior management to 'sell' the changes in a video and issue the T-shirts – but it will not do much for the mental well-being of employees in a change or reorganisation! The pace of change for businesses is unlikely to slow in the new global economy and those which are to be successful will be those that manage the process effectively. The arguments and examples set out here provide some thoughts on how to secure a win–win situation in which change is successfully implemented while safeguarding the mental well-being of employees.

References

Gratton, L. (1997) Tomorrow people. *People Management*, 24 July.
Kim, W. C. & Mauborgue, R. (1997) Fair process: managing in the knowledge economy. *Harvard Business Review*, July–August.

CHAPTER 2

Legal aspects of mental health in the workplace

Denis D'Auria, Gillian Howard and Peter Verow

This chapter briefly reviews the key points of legal importance concerning mental health in the workplace. There have been some significant developments under both statute and case law that have placed clear responsibilities on employers in the workplace to protect employees from mental health problems and that have made them more responsible when recruiting staff and when dismissing staff who have or have had mental illness. Under the Disability Discrimination Act 1995 there are very clear duties on employers before rejecting job candidates with a history of mental illness to try to make reasonable adjustments to the workplace (see Box 2.1). This duty to make reasonable adjustments applies also to employees who develop mental health problems during their employment.

Box 2.1 The Farnsworth case
(*London Borough of Hammersmith and Fulham* v. *Farnsworth*)

In a case involving the previous mental health of a social worker, Ms Farnsworth, who was rejected by the London Borough of Hammersmith and Fulham Council for a post working with children with special needs because of an earlier history of clinical depression, the Employment Appeal Tribunal held that the employers had discriminated against her. They could have made reasonable adjustments such as placing her on a probationary period, supervising her closely during this period and monitoring her work and her absence record. In this case, it was the occupational health physician who recommended that the Council should not employ Ms Farnsworth because of her history of clinical depression. The Borough knew about this history because Ms Farnsworth had given her consent for the Borough to see her medical questionnaire and to have her medical history disclosed to them.

Pre-employment assessment

The purpose of pre-employment health evaluation has been set out in several publications (e.g. Health and Safety Executive, 1982). Both the content of and output from these procedures should be job related. Given a history of psychiatric ill health, whether paranoid schizophrenia or depression, it may be tempting to fabricate a reason to reject the applicant, but if this is done without sufficient reason the employer's obligations under the Disability Discrimination Act 1995 are unlikely to be met.

When people have recovered from a mental illness, they are generally encouraged by their physicians and psychiatrists to return to the world of work, to function as before. The obstacles facing such people are immense and it is not surprising that some fail to disclose their history of mental ill health. They may not be lying. The questionnaire may simply not ask the question in the most appropriate terms; or perhaps an applicant may not have understood or have been given the full facts, or may simply deny them. Lying, however, if it occurs, and if it is material to the job, may serve 'as some other substantial reason' for dismissal under section 98(1)(b) of the Employment Rights Act 1996 (see also Box 2.2 and *Walton* v. *TAC Construction Materials*).

Box 2.2 The O'Brien case
(*O'Brien* v. *The Prudential Assurance Company Ltd*)

O'Brien applied for a job with the Prudential Assurance Company as a district agent. His job was to visit people in their homes. His prior psychiatric history included several hospital stays. At the time of his application he had not seen his doctor for four years, apart from consultations regarding minor illnesses. The pre-employment medical questionnaire asked about prior serious illnesses. The examining medical officer asked whether he had ever consulted a psychiatrist or has a nervous or mental disorder. O'Brien denied that he had, as he knew he would not get the job if he admitted this. The employers later confirmed this to be so. He proved an able employee but when he applied for life assurance with the company, he gave consent to the release of a medical report which showed that years earlier he had had schizophrenia. Despite the recommendations of a junior manager, he was referred to the principal medical adviser, who later recommended dismissal without further medical evidence being obtained. The Employment Tribunal and Employment Appeal Tribunal upheld the dismissal as fair on the grounds that Prudential's medical advice was that he would not have been employed as a district agent with that kind of mental history and that his lying on his application form and at his medical pre-employment interview was a significant and material deceit such as to justify his summary dismissal. However, it is likely now that under the Disability Discrimination Act 1995 (see below), such a dismissal could be held to be unlawful (for which there is no cap on compensation).

The responses to medical questionnaires are confidential and should not be disclosed to human resources managers. If the material is stored on computer or in manual records, this would be a breach of the first principle of the Data Protection Act 1998. It would also breach the implied duty of mutual trust and confidence that is a fundamental term of the employment contract. It is also arguably a breach of the Misrepresentation Act 1976 (*McNally* v. *Welltrade International Ltd*). Each case is, of course, actionable.

After the scandals of the early 1960s, information about prior mental illness was commonly sought from applicants for certain posts. This was usually part of the general application form and frequently created difficulty for applicants. However, human resources managers and personnel officers can ask questions that do not undermine medical confidentiality, such as 'Have you seen your doctor in the past five years'?

It is not acceptable for a lay person to ask whether the applicant has been admitted to a psychiatric hospital or has had a nervous disorder. As well as being frequently asked at interview, health questions are often added to general application forms processed by the human resource rather than occupational health department. The applicant should be made aware of which department will process the information at the beginning *and not the end* of the form. Suggestions that misleading information on these medical questionnaires will make any contract void or lead to instant dismissal are either meaningless or indefensible.

It should be noted that the obtaining, storing, using, disclosing or otherwise of any health information is regarded as 'sensitive' data under section 2 of the Data Protection Act 1998 and, as such, express informed written consent must be obtained from the job applicant before such information can be gathered. Part 1 of the Code of Practice published under the Data Protection Act covers the gathering of sensitive health data and advises that informed consent will not have been obtained if there is any duress on the job applicant to give consent. Another part of the Code of Practice specifically covers medical records.

Preventing mental health problems

Statutory liability

There is no specific legislative guidance on stress and mental health, although the Health and Safety Executive (HSE) (1995) has published guidance on stress at work. Employers have a general duty to ensure, as far as is reasonably practicable, the health, safety and welfare of the workforce (section 2 of the Health and Safety at Work etc. Act 1974). This duty applies to both physical and mental health: the Act is concerned with both, as it defines 'personal injury' to include 'any disease and any impairment of a person's physical or mental condition' (section 53).

Risks, including those arising from stress in the workplace, must also be assessed under the Management of Health and Safety at Work Regulations 1999. The Health and Safety Executive's guidance leaflet on first-aid measures and guidance note (Health and Safety Executive, 1988, 1993, 1995, 2001 respectively) are indicative of the seriousness attached to stress and mental health. Each will be of use in future litigation to establish a 'date of knowledge'.

Common law liability

The court in *Walker* v. *Northumberland County Council* (detailed in Chapter 4, Box 4.2, p. 30) concluded that management of the risk of psychiatric damage arising from the amount or character of an employee's work is part of the duty of care owed to the employee. Walker was successful because the defendants failed to provide a reasonably safe working system and failed to protect him from risks which, after an initial mental breakdown and his subsequent return to work, had become reasonably foreseeable. The key issue is reasonable foreseeability, which is a difficult burden for the claimant. *Walker* was successful because his breakdown had placed his employers on notice that his work could adversely affect on his mental health.

While the Walker case suggests that liability is easier to prove for a second episode of mental ill health, there are two important points to note. First, given the growing awareness of stress at work, it cannot be assumed that liability will continue to attach only to the second attack. Second, employers will be reasonably expected to reduce pressures in the workplace, where they are within the employer's control. These will include not only ergonomic and environmental factors, since these are capable of systematic assessment, as required under the Management Regulations 1992, but also behavioural aspects, such as harassment. These are often associated with problems with the style of management, such as inconsistency, indifference and bullying.

Likely defences to future litigation may include systematic review of sickness absence records, clinical investigation of workplace stress and the adoption of stress management measures, such as minimum periods of holiday.

The Court of Appeal gave useful guidance on when employers will be held liable for negligence in causing stress-related illness or injury and what measures they should adopt to avoid liability (*Sutherland and Hatton* v. *Somerset County Council* and three other joined appeals). The points below are a summary of what the Court of Appeal held in these cases and of the practical propositions set out by the Court of Appeal for the guidance of courts concerned with this type of claim in future.

- There are no special control mechanisms applying to claims for psychiatric (or physical) illness or injury arising from the stress of doing the work the employee is required to do. The ordinary principles of employer's liability apply.
- The threshold question is whether this kind of harm to this particular employee was *reasonably foreseeable*. This has two components: (a) an injury to health (as distinct from occupational stress) which (b) is attributable to stress at work (as distinct from other factors).
- *Foreseeability* depends upon what the employer knows (or ought reasonably to know) about the individual employee. Because of its nature, mental disorder is harder to foresee than physical injury, but may be easier to foresee in a known individual than in the population at large. Employers are usually entitled to assume that the employee can withstand the normal pressures of the job unless they know of some particular problem or vulnerability (i.e. staff who feel under stress at work should tell their employers and give them a chance to do something about it).
- The test is the same whatever the employment: there are no occupations which should be regarded as intrinsically dangerous to mental health.
- Factors likely to be relevant in answering the threshold question relate to the nature and extent of the work done by the employee: 'Is the workload much more than is normal for the particular job?', 'Is the work particularly intellectually or emotionally demanding for this employee?', 'Are the demands being made of this employee unreasonable when compared with the demands made of others in the same or comparable jobs, or are there signs that others doing this job are suffering harmful levels of stress?', 'Is there an abnormal level of sickness or absenteeism in the same job or the same department?'
- Further questions will relate to signs from the employee of impending harm to health: 'Has he a particular problem or vulnerability?', 'Has he already suffered from illness attributable to stress at work?', 'Have there recently been frequent or prolonged absences which are uncharacteristic of him?', 'Is there reason to think that these are attributable to stress at work, for example because of complaints or warnings from him or others?'
- Employers are generally entitled to take what they are told by an employee at face value, unless they have good reason to think to the contrary. They do not generally have to make searching enquiries of the employee or seek permission to make further enquiries of his medical advisers.
- To trigger a duty to take steps, the indications of impending harm to health arising from stress at work must be plain enough for any

reasonable employer to realise that he or she should do something about it.

- Employers are in breach of duty only if they have failed to take the steps which are reasonable in the circumstances, bearing in mind the magnitude of the risk of harm occurring, the gravity of the harm which may occur, the costs and practicability of preventing it, and the justifications for running the risk.

- The size and scope of the employer's operation, its resources and the demands it faces are relevant in deciding what is reasonable; these include the interests of other employees and the need to treat them fairly, for example in any redistribution of duties.

- An employer can reasonably be expected only to take steps which are likely to do some good: the court is likely to need expert evidence on this.

- An employer who offers a confidential advice service, with referral to appropriate counselling or treatment services, is unlikely to be found in breach of duty.

- If the only reasonable and effective step would have been to dismiss or demote the employee, the employer will not be in breach of duty in allowing a willing employee to continue in the job.

- In all cases, therefore, it is necessary to identify the steps which the employer both could and should have taken before finding the employer in breach of his or her duty of care.

- The claimant must show that that breach of duty has caused or materially contributed to the harm suffered. It is not enough to show that occupational stress has caused the harm.

- Where the harm suffered has more than one cause, the employer should pay only for that proportion of the harm suffered which is attributable to his or her wrongdoing, unless the harm is truly indivisible.

- The assessment of damages will take account of any pre-existing disorder or vulnerability and of the chance that the claimant would have succumbed to a stress-related disorder in any event.

Liability in contract

A breach of contract may occur when an employer exercises an express discretionary contractual power to require employees to work additional hours, for example in relation to overtime and hours of work, when it contravenes that employer's implied contractual duty to take reasonable care of the health and safety of its employees.

The Working Time Regulations 1998 now restrict most workers to a limit of 48 hours in any seven-day period averaged over 17 weeks. Workers can opt out by giving their written consent to work longer hours and certain categories of workers are exempt from the 48-hour limit.

A fundamental implied duty of trust and confidence means that employees should not be subject to abuse or harassment by their employers or co-workers in respect of whom the employer may be vicariously liable. Employers must not prevent employees' attempts to fulfil their contractual obligations. This duty may be breached, for example, if an employer fails to provide sufficient support and resources for an appointee to carry out a job. Remedies can be sought from the civil courts and industrial tribunals for constructive dismissal.

Confidentiality

Confidence in the occupational physician and trust that an employee may speak frankly are essential to the relationship. Although it is clearly an ethical obligation, the law has developed in a haphazard manner and the precise nature of any obligation of confidence remains uncertain (see para. 3.1 of the Law Commission report no. 110, 1981; Jones, 1970). An examination of case law on breach of confidence suggests certain principles. First, courts will intervene where information is confidential and not public knowledge. Second, courts will act in situations where information is disclosed in circumstances where confidentiality might have been expected. Third, they will act where that confidentiality should be protected in the public interest (*W* v. *Egdell*).

The difficulty lies not in the obligation of medical confidentiality but in deciding when disclosure is justified. Where a court order or statutory obligation exists, there is no difficulty. In other circumstances that affect the occupational physician, disclosure may be necessary in the public interest. This often used to concern the disclosure of crime, but public interest is now interpreted more widely (*Lion Laboratories* v. *Evans*).

Despite recent judgements, there remains a host of uncertainty; in such instances resort should be made to guidance of the General Medical Council (GMC). The GMC permits disclosure where:

- the patient or legal adviser gives written informed consent
- information is shared with others involved in the patient care
- it is undesirable on medical grounds to seek patient consent, when information may be given to a close relative
- disclosure to a third party other than a relative would be in the patient's best interests
- it is necessary to comply with statutory requirements
- it is required by court order
- it is in the public interest
- it is required for a research project approved by a recognised ethical committee.

Patients dissatisfied with the outcome of a complaint to the GMC have no appeal but it is open to them to seek redress from the courts – in the Privy Council – but only on a point of law.

Access to Medical Reports Act 1988

The Act concerns reports prepared for insurance or employment purposes by physicians who have or have had clinical care of the patient. Rights of access are well known but the reporting physician is permitted to withhold the report or part from the patient if it would cause, inter alia, serious harm to the patient's physical or mental health or that of others. Patients must nonetheless be told it is to be withheld so that they can consent to it being supplied to the party originating the request.

The Act provides that a complaint of a breach of the Act may be made to a county court, which may order the employer, insurance company or doctor to comply. This may bring the doctor to the notice of the GMC.

Access to Health Records Act 1990

Since 1 November 1991, there is a statutory right of access to health records made in connection with the care of the individual. Once again, difficulties may arise where psychiatric ill health is concerned, despite the modern tendency towards openness in discussions of such matters. Under section 5 of the Act, a doctor is permitted to withhold the record or part of the record where, for example, disclosure is likely to cause serious harm to the physical or mental health of the patient or of any other individual.

This Act has been repealed by the Data Protection Act 1998.

Data Protection Act 1998

This Act came into force on 1 March 2000 and encompasses both computerised and manual records. The Act defines two categories of persons. The data subject is, of course, the patient. The data controller is the person responsible for processing and determining the purpose of holding and storing the data. This is usually the employer but may on occasion be the individual physician.

It is a criminal offence to process data unless the employer has fulfilled the notification procedure (previously called registration). Processing includes organising, consulting, using, disclosing and destroying the data.

The Act identifies two subcategories of data. Personal data are data through which it is possible to identify a living individual. Sensitive personal data include 'information as to [the] physical or mental health and condition of the data subject', as set out in section 2(e). These data must be processed in accordance with the data protection principles as set out in section 4 and Schedule I, Part 1 of the Act. The most important and probably relevant of these is that both personal and sensitive personal data may be processed only fairly and lawfully.

There are many pitfalls in the Act and we must await case law before seeing how its interpretation will fashion occupational health practice in the real world.

Human Rights Act 1998

The Human Rights Act came into effect on 2 October 2000 and incorporates into law the European Convention on Human Rights and Fundamental Freedoms, which was ratified by the UK on 8 March 1951 and came into force on 23 September 1953. Until the passing of this Act, there was no right of individual petition and no mandatory acceptance of the Convention's jurisdiction in UK courts.

Section 1 of the Act provides that articles of the Convention are now given effect in domestic law. Section 3 requires primary and subordinate legislation to be read and given effect in a way that is compatible with the Convention.

Article 8 of the Convention confers a right to respect for privacy and medical data, and maintenance of confidentiality has been held to fall within its scope (*MSB* v. *Sweden*). The courts have so far taken a pragmatic approach to the granting of applications under the Act. However, it is likely that the Act will be used to protect the area of confidentiality, which, legally speaking, has been in a chaotic state for a long time.

Emergency treatment in the workplace

While a full understanding of the proper use of compulsory admission can be obtained only from extensive clinical experience, on rare occasions the occupational physician may need to be aware of the general conditions governing it.

The most likely matter of concern is an acute psychotic reaction where an individual may be placing him- or herself or co-workers in danger. The appropriate management is an emergency order for assessment under section 4 of the Mental Health Act 1983, which is usually completed by the family doctor, but may be used in other situations when there is insufficient time to gain the opinion of an approved doctor, who could complete a section 2 order. An application must be made by an approved social worker or the nearest relative and must be supported by the medical recommendation of a doctor, who need not be approved under section 12 of the Act. Admission must take place within 24 hours.

Under section 136 of the Act, a police constable who finds somebody appearing to be suffering from a mental disorder in a public place may take that person to a place of safety, usually a police station or hospital. The individual must be in immediate need of care or control; it must be in the individual's best interests or for the further protection of other persons.

Unfair dismissal

The leading case on the question of dismissals on the grounds of ill health (*East Lindsey District Council* v. *Daubney*) is outlined in Box 2.3.

The employer is expected to act fairly, considering the nature of the job, the size of the business and the nature of the employee's illness. Psychiatric illness is often of long duration and there are likely to be relapses. As a general rule, medical evidence must be sought to assess the potential for return to work and the likely capability of the employee. A consultation must take place between the manager and the employee to assess the likelihood of a return to work, to warn the employee that his or her job is in jeopardy, to ascertain the true medical position, and to allow consideration of options such as making adjustments to the employee's job (reduced hours and/or duties) or transferring the employee to a different job.

If the individual is being interviewed in a disciplinary context, it is wise to give physicians or psychiatrists the opportunity to comment on whether or not the patient is fit for disciplinary interview. The majority of employees clearly understand the nature of the difficulties and can participate in proceedings. Their situation would be substantially improved if outstanding issues were resolved. For this reason, it is important that psychiatric patients are at least represented by a union representative or work colleague and this right is now enshrined in statute (sections 10–12 of the Employment Relations Act 1999).

Box 2.3 The leading case for unfair dismissal on the grounds of ill health (*East Lindsey District Council* v. *Daubney*)

A surveyor employed by the East Lindsey District Council was dismissed after long periods of absence due to anxiety. The personnel director sought medical advice from the district community physician, who wrote that the employee was unfit and should be retired on medical grounds. This was implemented without indicating to the employee that his job was in jeopardy or allowing him to seek his own doctor's advice.

Disability Discrimination Act 1995

Under the Act, a mental impairment is defined as one 'resulting from or consisting of a mental illness, only if the illness is a clinically well recognised illness'. It is likely that any mental illness classified under the DSM or ICD classifications would be considered to be 'well recognised'. Addictive behaviours and behavioural and antisocial disorders are not.

The Act's protection applies to those disabilities which have lasted or are likely to last for 12 months or more. In addition, they must have 'a substantial and adverse effect' upon the carrying out of at least one of the normal day-to-day activities listed in Schedule 1 of the Act. These include 'memory or ability to concentrate, learn or understand', but do not necessarily apply only to the workplace.

One of the earliest successful applications to an industrial tribunal concerned chronic fatigue syndrome. It was successful as it is defined by the World Health Organization (WHO) as a separate neurological disorder and is recognised by the Royal Colleges of Psychiatrists, Physicians and General Practitioners as a seriously debilitating and genuine disorder. Whether it is psychiatric or neurological is not at issue – there is a resulting disability.

Whether or not a person with a clinically well-recognised mental illness is an applicant or an employee, employers are under an obligation to 'make reasonable adjustments to the workplace'. Reasonable adjustments can focus on the individual, such as requiring him or her to take a holiday, rest away from work, time off for treatment, training or redeployment, avoiding shift work or stressful tasks, the introduction of a mentoring system, and arrangements for a visiting psychiatrist or for supervision by the occupational health service.

The Employment Appeal Tribunal (EAT) in the case of *Morgan* v. *Staffordshire University* (2002) held that tribunals will expect a more focused diagnosis than 'stress', 'depression' or 'anxiety' before they will be prepared to accept that the individual has a mental illness. In this case, Mrs Morgan's general practitioner had certified that she was suffering from 'stress'. The EAT held that:

'As the WHO ICD does not use such terms, without qualification, and there is no general acceptance of such loose terms, it is not the case that some loose description such as "anxiety", "stress" or "depression" of itself will suffice.... Whilst the words "anxiety", "stress" and "depression" could be dug at intervals out of the copies of the medical notes put before the Tribunal, it is not the case that their occasional use, even by medical men, will, without further explanation, amount to proof of a mental impairment within the Act, still less as its proof as at some particular time. Even G.P.s, we suspect, sometimes use such terms without having a technical meaning in mind and none of the notes, without further explanation, can be read as

Box 2.4 The Kapadia case
(*Kapadia* v. *London Borough of Lambeth*)

Mr Kapadia, an accountant at Lambeth, had been diagnosed by his doctor as having reactive depression. He had been in and out of hospital and had received counselling for over two years. He was ultimately dismissed as being medically unfit to perform his duties. He brought a claim for unlawful discrimination for a reason relating to his disability. The employment tribunal found that his mental impairment did not have a substantial impact upon the carrying out of normal day-to-day activities and therefore dismissed his claim.

The Court of Appeal found that the employment tribunal had erred in law in finding that the applicant's mental impairment did not have a substantial adverse effect on his normal day-to-day activities in circumstances in which there was uncontested medical evidence that his anxiety, neuroses and depression would have had such an effect but for the fact that he had received medical treatment.

The employment tribunal was obliged to come to the conclusion that the applicant had proved his case given that there was direct evidence from two medical experts that there was an underlying disability which was concealed by the medical treatment. There was no contrary expert medical evidence or challenge to the factual bases of those opinions.

intending to indicate the presence of a classified or classifiable mental illness, either after the exacerbating events of the assault proceedings were over or at all. Indeed, the notes of the Professor of Psychiatry, possibly the most authoritative although speaking of a distant time, suggest its absence. There was no evidence from any doctor to explain what he had meant at the time his note was made, nor to assert that Mrs Morgan was at any time mentally impaired within the Act. Without our here setting out further extracts from the WHO ICD, we notice that the work shows at many parts of its classification that specific symptoms, often required to be manifest over a minimum specified period or with a minimum specified frequency, are required if a claimant relies upon falling within it.'

Finally, it is not for the tribunals to decide whether or not someone has a mental illness where there is clear medical evidence (Box 2.4).

References

Health and Safety Executive (1982) *Guidance Note MS 20 – Pre-employment Health Screening*. London: HSE.
— (1988) *Mental Health in the Workplace*. London: HSE.
— (1993) *Mental Distress at Work*. London: HSE.
— (1995) *Stress at Work*. London: HSE.
— (2001) *Tackling Work-Related Stress*. London: HSE.

Jones, G. (1970) Restitution of benefits obtained in breach of another's confidence. *LQR*, **86**, 463.

Law Commission (1981) *Breach of Confidence*, report no. 110, cmd 8388. London: HMSO.

Cases

East Lindsey District Council v. *Daubney* [1977] IRLR 181.

Kapadia v. *London Borough of Lambeth* [2000] IRLR 699.

Lion Laboratories v. *Evans* [1984] 2 All ER 417 at 433.

London Borough of Hammersmith and Fulham v. *Farnsworth* [2000] IRLR 691.

McNally v. *Welltrade International Ltd* [1978] IRLR 497.

Morgan v. *Staffordshire University* [2002] IRLR 190.

MSB v. *Sweden* 23 EHRR 313, European Court of Human Rights.

O'Brien v. *The Prudential Assurance Company Ltd* [1979] IRLR 140.

Sutherland and Hatton v. *Somerset County Council; Barker* v. *Somerset County Council; Bishop* v. *Baker Refractories Ltd; Jones* v. *Sandwell Metropolitan Borough Council* [2002] EWCA Civ. 76; CA Civil Division.

W v. *Edgell* [1990] 1 All ER 835 at 846 (CA).

Walker v. *Northumberland County Council* [1995] IRLR 35; QB.

Walton v. *TAC Construction Materials* [1981] IRLR 357.

CHAPTER 3

Risk management approach to mental health: the London Electricity case study

Anne Margaret Samuel

Introduction

London Electricity has taken a holistic approach to the management of mental ill health at work by ensuring that it forms part of an overall health and safety risk management strategy. This approach aims to destigmatise mental illness while ensuring that its impact on human behaviour is taken fully into account in the management of health and safety risks. Consequently the management of mental health forms one of the modules of the health risk management programme developed by London Electricity called 'Fit For Work'.

This programme requires the company to take an 'upstream', preventive approach to managing occupational health risks, rather than a more traditional 'downstream', reactive approach, which relies on treatment, rehabilitation and ill-health retirement to manage occupational ill health. However, to be successful, the preventive approach requires the right culture in which to thrive and, critically, it must have the commitment and support of senior managers. This is not only to ensure that the right values and behaviours are exhibited by senior managers and those who report to them, but also to ensure that employees are encouraged to attend training sessions designed to inform them about the potential occupational health and safety risks to which they are exposed.

The rationale behind this approach is to reduce costs, in terms of both the suffering of individual employees and the 'bottom line' of business finances. During training for managers, inverted pyramids (Figure 3.1) are used to drive home the point about how to manage mental ill health at work. Clearly there are also cost implications in successfully implementing a health risk management programme such as Fit For Work. Staff have to be released for awareness training and provision has to be made for any necessary control measures emanating from the risk assessments. These costs are very apparent to managers because they have to budget for them upfront. However, when compared

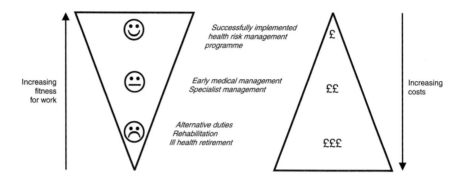

Figure 3.1 The costs of managing mental health.

with the less visible, but no less real, costs of medical management, ill health retirement and litigation, the costs of implementing a health risk management programme appear a prudent investment.

The Fit for Work programme

The Fit for Work programme consists of six modules covering: chemical, physical, manual handling; display screen equipment (DSE); new or expectant mothers; ergonomics; risk management; and mental health. All modules follow the same principles: hazards are identified, risks are assessed and control measures are identified.

The mental health module has themed leaflets to support it, including ones entitled *Understanding Stress* and *Post Traumatic Stress* and another explaining London Electricity's employee support programme. The module assists with the identification of potential 'stress' hazards, the assessment of how likely they are to cause mental ill health and the implementation of measures necessary to avoid risk as far is reasonably practicable. Perhaps the most important step in this process is risk assessment and, in terms of managing mental health, assessing particular task requirements in terms of their physical and mental demands, as shown in Figure 3.2. Ensuring that these demands match the skills and aptitude of the employee who is expected to do the job is of crucial importance in preventing both physical and mental health problems.

Risk assessment

No one is better placed to assess the employee in his or her working environment than the line manager or supervisor. The line manager is

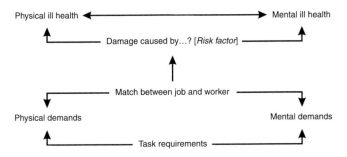

Figure 3.2 Model of risk assessment used in London Electricity's Fit For Work programme.

required to take the necessary steps through the relevant Fit For Work modules to manage the physical risks associated with the job, which can, and often do, lead to stress problems if left uncontrolled. The Fit For Work mental health module develops this into psychosocial hazards and is targeted at the management of potential mental health problems. It aims to help managers to identify early warning signs, including those associated with alcohol and drug misuse.

The nub of the module is encouraging the supervisor or manager to 'know the person', recognising whether a gap has developed between the expected and actual performance of the employee and doing something about it. The most common explanations for such a gap are 'being a square peg in a round hole' (mismatch of employee to job), family or money problems, personality clashes or poor management style. It is critical to ensure that supervisors and managers are well trained in conducting sensitive interviews with their staff, particularly in knowing when not to probe too deeply and to involve specialist support, such as occupational health staff. Essentially, the risk management strategy for mental health at London Electricity is ergonomics based, as the following case study demonstrates.

Case study

In 1997, at London Electricity there was an increasing number of referrals to the occupational health department for musculoskeletal and stress symptoms among a group of staff responsible for undertaking routine DSE work and dealing with customer enquiries. In light of this trend, the occupational health department, along with London Electricity's ergonomics and occupational physiotherapy providers (COPE) carried out a survey of 110 employees in this group. Having carried out

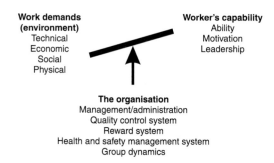

Figure 3.3 Functional mismatch: the balance between work demands and the worker's capability, within the organisation.

thorough DSE assessments, a Role Interventional Assessment Tool (RIAT), which was designed by COPE, was used to identify potential areas of functional mismatch (Figure 3.3) among this group.

A questionnaire was administered to the staff through face-to-face interview, analysed and the results presented to management. Over the next two months many of the recommendations made by the occupational health department to address functional mismatch were adopted. Although it was possible to readminister the questionnaire to only a subsample of the group (50 employees), a comparison of outcomes on two of the RIAT measures, namely motivation and work demands, showed the effectiveness of the intervention. The question posed to employees about motivation was 'How often do you find your work interesting?' The responses are shown in Figure 3.4. The question

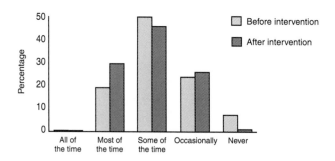

Figure 3.4 Comparison of outcomes on the motivation Role Intervention Assessment Tool (RIAT) measure ('How often do you find your work interesting?'), before ($n = 110$) and two months after ($n = 50$) the intervention by the occupational health department at London Electricity to address functional mismatch.

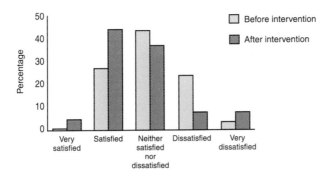

Figure 3.5 Comparison of outcomes on the work demands Role Intervention Assessment Tool (RIAT) measure ('Overall, how do you feel about your job content?'), before (n = 110) and two months after (n = 50) the intervention by the occupational health department at London Electricity to address functional mismatch.

relating to work demands was 'Overall, how do you feel about your job content?' The response is shown in Figure 3.5.

Two interventions appeared to explain the improved satisfaction rating over the two-month period for both parameters (motivation and work demands). They were:

(1) the introduction of a filtering system for telephone calls so that customers were directed to staff with the appropriate expertise in dealing with their queries (motivation);

(2) the introduction of a more flexible 'break system' which was acceptable to both management and staff, and brief but effective 'energizer exercises' at the workstation (work demands).

Conclusion

London Electricity takes a holistic approach towards the management of mental health at work by making it a critical component of the Fit For Work health risk management programme, which is based on ergonomic principles. In addition to risk management, the occupational health department has close links with a clinical psychologist and his or her team. They provide change management training to all managers and provide a confidential employee support programme for London Electricity employees. The programme is closely linked with the occupational health department and acts as a safety net, underpinning other control measures, and effectively 'closes the loop' on the management of mental health at work.

CHAPTER 4

Mental well-being in the workplace: building the business case

Noeleen Doherty

Introduction

More than 25 million people in the UK engage in paid employment. The protection of employees' physical health has been a priority for many years but safeguarding the *mental* well-being of the workforce has received far less attention. Until recently, in most organisations, the employer's role in dealing with mental health issues has been poorly defined, with little coherent guidance or evidence regarding good practice.

There is an ethical and a moral case for the management of mental well-being within the organisational context. It has been argued (Jones & Lowndes, 1997) that organisations should implement a policy of good human relations which treats all employees with respect and trust and supports their individual development needs. The benefit is said to accrue from the generation of the reciprocal commitment required for excellent performance and hence organisational success. However, this mutuality of interest between company and employee can be challenged. The bulk of evidence suggests that few organisations are, in practice, proactive and preventive in their approach to managing mental well-being. Most companies are entirely reactive to mental illness when it occurs and, even then, it usually features on the business agenda only when attempts are made to address issues such as sickness absence and the resultant costs to the business.

Commercial organisations, of necessity, focus on financial outcomes and, if mental well-being is to be addressed in the workplace, there is a requirement for a business case which focuses on business objectives and which helps to fulfil business needs. There is a fundamental need to justify why mental well-being is important to businesses and a growing pressure to provide data to show the financial impact of various options so that a cost–benefit analysis can be undertaken. Building the business case is standard practice for any proposed investment and health initiatives in the workplace should be no different. Assembling valid financial and cost-oriented data is the cornerstone of such a business case and must therefore be the starting point for those seeking to place mental well-being on the management agenda.

The costs of mental ill health

The headline cost of mental ill health to business is often shown as the sick pay bill. However, this neglects 'hidden' costs of absenteeism, such as those associated with lost productivity, reduced work performance, hiring replacement labour and the costs in management time of adjusting work schedules, completing statutory forms and so on. Additional costs to business include increased insurance premiums, medical severance or early retirement costs and, increasingly in the UK, litigation. Combining costs in this way gives a truer picture of the impact of mental illness on an organisation. The main elements contributing to the overall cost of mental ill health to business are summarised in Box 4.1.

Estimates of the overall costs of mental ill health in the UK are based on published data from a variety of different sources and on information not gathered primarily for this purpose. There is consequential variation in the figures arrived at but there is consistency in the general scale of the financial burden. Taylor (1995), in the *Financial Times*, has reported that, at any one time, 2.2 million people suffer from work-related ill health (physical and mental) and that this costs the economy between £4 billion and £9 billion per annum. Sickness absence surveys (Muir, 1994; CBI, 1995) have shown that 30–35% of employee sick leave in the UK is said to be related to stress, anxiety or depression. The Department of Health (1995) estimated that 91 million working days each year are lost through stress-related illness, at a cost to industry of £3.7 billion. It is generally accepted that approximately three in ten employees will have a mental health problem, and that this will account for some 80 million lost working days each year; taking account of the resultant

---

Box 4.1 The cost of mental ill health to business

- Sick pay
- Lost productivity
- Additional labour/overtime
- Administration costs
- Increasing insurance premiums
- Medical severance or early retirement on health grounds
- Litigation costs

sickness absence, labour turnover, poor performance and accidents at work, the annual cost to industry is said to be £5.3 billion (Banham, 1992).

The costs of litigation

These estimated costs are very significant but do not include costs associated with the risk of litigation. Personal injury claims against employers for damage to mental health have been uncommon in the UK until recently but the number is rising rapidly and this risk must now feature in any analysis of cost and benefit. The landmark case was that of *Walker v. Northumberland County Council* and this legal action has raised the profile of mental well-being for business throughout the UK. Details are given in Box 4.2 (see also Welch, 1996).

Further evidence of the growing trend in claims and damages against companies is provided by data gathered about insurance and compensation claims. For example, Unum Provident (2002) indicated that changes in work patterns in the UK had resulted in a 50% increase in claims for compensation arising from mental and psychological problems between 1995 and 2001. The Trades Union Congress (TUC) calculated that, in 1994, members of affiliated trade unions were awarded a total of £355 million in legal damages after suffering injury or ill health as a result of their work (Institute of Personnel and Development, 1995).

Although the sources may be disparate and have different cost bases, there appears to be a considerable amount of data and convincing

---

Box 4.2 The Walker case: setting a precedent

The case of John Walker, a social worker with Northumberland County Council, has drawn much attention to the importance of mental well-being in the work context. Walker suffered a nervous breakdown in 1986, having complained of overwork due to under-staffing and lack of administrative support. He returned to work after four months, but suffered a further mental breakdown brought on by stress due to his 'impossible workload'. He retired on medical grounds in May 1988. A High Court judge ruled that the County Council was responsible for causing his breakdown, as it was in breach of its duty of care to Walker by continuing to employ him following the first breakdown without providing additional support. The judge ruled that there was sufficient evidence to indicate that, had the Council provided adequate assistance on his return to work, Walker would probably not have suffered a second breakdown. The Council agreed to settle before appeal and agreed a record £175,000 in damages.

Box 4.3 Barclays Bank

A survey of 4600 managers in Barclays Bank indicated that nearly half felt insecure about their jobs, 19% worked up to or over 25 hours a week overtime and a quarter had received medical treatment for stress-related illnesses over the past five years. As a result, Barclays have contracted a counselling service as one mechanism to help employees to cope (Welch, 1996).

---

evidence to suggest that, when things go wrong, impaired mental well-being can be very expensive for companies. The undeniable message is that mental ill health among employees is potentially a major financial consideration in the balance sheet.

Promoting mental well-being

The damaging effects to a business of the costs of mental ill health need to be managed, but there are also benefits associated with promoting mental well-being in the workplace. The objective of promoting well-being is to encourage all employees to optimise performance by creating a healthy environment. At the level of the individual employee this can be achieved through health education programmes, health screening and other targeted interventions. Such programmes can have a number of aims. They include enhancing the image of the company as one which cares for employee well-being. This may have 'spin-off' effects, such as higher staff retention, improved motivation and the creation of a good corporate image. These programmes also aim to reduce the costs of medical care and to enhance productivity by cutting absenteeism and its associated costs. Some organisations have recognised this and, as in the case of Barclays Bank (Box 4.3), the burgeoning cost of medical treatment has prompted them to take action to address mental well-being issues.

Calculating the benefits of an intervention

The assumption is often made that, in addition to reducing tangible costs, health education, screening and intervention programmes will help already healthy workers to be more productive. However, the correlation between health programmes and increased motivation or performance is often difficult to demonstrate. Since individual health behaviour is a complex mix of social and economic factors it is difficult to attribute changes in such behaviour directly to the use of health promotion or intervention programmes. This renders the financial

> **Box 4.4** The Post Office
>
> Specific initiatives designed to reduce work-related risks posed to employees within the Post Office resulted in financial benefits. A programme designed to address absence caused by post-traumatic stress resulted in cost savings of £100 000 per annum. The programme reduced trauma-related sickness absence by 50%. Additionally, a programme targeting general stress-related problems reduced stress-related sickness absence by 32% and was calculated to save £115,000 per annum.

calculation of savings or benefits for this type of proactive approach problematic. Few organisations have fully analysed the cost–benefits of health promotion programmes, and in particular of programmes which focus on mental health. Gaps in this information undermine the ability to include it as a persuasive element in the business case.

One organisation which has attempted to calculate the cost–benefit of interventions is the Post Office (formerly Consignia) (Box 4.4) (Doherty & Tyson, 1998). This is one of the few examples of this type of cost–benefit analysis because of the difficulties in showing direct correlations between programmes and interventions and bottom line results.

The management of costs and potential costs appears to be the major driver for a business case which addresses mental well-being as a key management objective. However, there are dangers in taking an approach which focuses entirely on the bottom line. The current dearth of coherent methods for calculating the cost–benefit of programmes which promote mental well-being inevitably leads to reactive measures. This type of retrospective damage limitation is intuitively less desirable and work is urgently required to properly cost proactive measures.

Conclusion

The current business environment is one of major organisational change at an accelerating pace. For both companies and individuals this has resulted in higher performance expectations within an increasingly insecure environment, and this provides fertile ground for potential mental health problems for employees. Business plans need to be regularly revised and success or failure often rests on the performance of a few key staff. Creating a dynamic environment in which success is nurtured relies on many factors, but in most modern companies, the people are seen a critical factor and safeguarding their well-being is a business imperative. However, many managers are ill equipped to cope with identifying the hazards and risks to mental well-being or the effects of mental ill health. Companies therefore need to address these threats to their staff and their profitability as part of their business planning. It may currently be difficult to quantify all of the costs and benefits in hard financial terms but that does not mean that they can be ignored, since to do so could have a major adverse long-term impact on the business.

Acknowledgement

The author acknowledges the support of the Health and Safety Executive in funding the research on which this chapter is based.

References

Banham, J. (1992) The costs of mental ill-health to business. In *Prevention of Mental Ill-health at Work: A Conference* (eds R. Jenkins & N. Coney), pp. 24–29. London: HMSO.

CBI (1995) *Managing Absence. CBI/Centre File Survey*. London: CBI.

Department of Health (1995) *ABC of Health Promotion in the Workplace. A Resource Pack for Employees*. London: Department of Health.

Doherty, N. & Tyson, S. (1998) *Mental Well-being in the Workplace. A Resource Pack for Management Training and Development*. Sudbury: HSE Books.

Institute of Personnel and Development (1995) *The IPD Guide on Occupational Health and Organisational Effectiveness*. London: Institute of Personnel and Development.

Jones, N. & Lowndes, S. N. (1997) The business case for occupational health services. In *The Corporate Healthcare Handbook* (ed. H. Kogan). London: Kogan Page.

Muir, J. (1994) Dealing with sickness absence. *Work Study*, **43** (5), 13–14.

Taylor, R. (1995) FT guide to health in the workplace (3): Healthy, wealthy and wise – a well workforce makes sound financial sense. *Financial Times*, 1 December, p. 3.

Unum Provident (2002) *The Living Insurer*. http://www.unumprovident.co.uk.

Welch, J. (1996) Stress ruling ups the stakes for employers. *People Management*, **2** (10), 13–15.

Case

Walker v. *Northumberland County Council* (1995) IRLR 35; QB.

Further reading

Department of Health (1995) *ABC of Health Promotion in the Workplace*. Health Information Service. London: Department of Health.

Kogan, H. (ed.) (1997) *The Corporate Healthcare Handbook*. London: Kogan Page.

CHAPTER 5

Developing a mental health policy: an outline

Ann Fingret

Introduction

This chapter, written from the perspective of an occupational health practitioner, presents an outline of where we are in relation to mental health in the workplace and a strategy for maintaining a healthy workforce. It is important to develop a structured approach to mental health in the workplace, not least because occupational health practitioners have frequently been guilty of interventions that may have been poorly researched and inappropriate. We have often been willing participants in unscientific approaches to resolving workplace problems.

As occupational health professionals, the research data that we have available is at odds with our personal experience in the workplace. This may be due to a lack of objectivity on our part or to fundamental flaws in the models applied. What is clear is that workplace stress is an increasing problem which produces many personal tragedies.

Prevailing cultures and management theories rely heavily on the commitment of the individual. One might think, therefore, that it is good business to nourish and preserve the *individual* employee. I have no doubt that if organisations are to survive and prosper they need to accept that paying attention to the psychological environment is essential. Occupational health practitioners have a part to play in ensuring that individual organisational environments are properly assessed and that appropriate interventions are prescribed and audited.

Incidence of work-related stress

In the 1990 Labour Force Survey in England and Wales (Office of Population Censuses and Surveys, 1992), 182 700 cases of stress related to work were reported. In the 1995 Survey of Self-Reported Work-Related Ill Health (Jones *et al*, 1998), 500 000 people in Great Britain reported that they were suffering from work-related stress, anxiety or depression, these causes collectively being second only to musculo-skeletal disorders. This suggests a 200% increase between 1990 and 1995, although this apparent increase may be due to better recognition or greater currency (Smith, 2000).

A survey of 500 members of the Institute of Directors in 1998 showed that 40% considered stress to be a big problem in their organisation (Smith, 2000).

The Bristol Stress and Health at Work Study used a random community sample to estimate the scale of occupational stress. Of the respondents, 10% reported that they were not stressed at all; 25–30% were mildly stressed; 40–45% reported moderate stress; and 15–20% described themselves as very stressed (Smith, 2000).

Absence for mental ill health and associated illness is estimated as 80 million working days (15% and 26% of all absence for men and women, respectively), at an estimated cost of £5.3 billion per year. However, the true cost of mental health problems to an organisation goes far beyond that of sickness absence and includes the impact of stress-related performance problems in those who are not off sick.

Occupational medicine practitioners have only slowly begun to address mental health problems in the workplace. A few landmarks of the developing interest are listed in Table 5.1. Although the list is undoubtedly idiosyncratic, it does follow the parallel development of management and occupational health responses to mental health problems.

The practice of occupational medicine has changed in response to these workplace transformations. This is borne out by a 1997 Faculty of Occupational Medicine survey which confirmed that psychological issues now take up a major part of the occupational physician's time

Table 5.1 Landmarks of the developing interest in occupational mental health

Year	Landmark
1914–18	Observations of health and performance in munitions workers
1939–45	The psychological assessment of mentally ill servicemen
1966	Formation of the Occupational Mental Health Discussion Group
1970 to date	The work of Cary Cooper at UMIST
1974	Health and Safety at Work Act
1990	The Health and Safety Executive publishes *Mental Health at Work*
1992	Management of Health and Safety at Work etc. Act
1994	*The Health of the Nation*
1994	*Walker* v. *Northumbria County Council*
1995	The Health and Safety Executive publishes *Stress at Work Guidelines*
1997	Disability Discrimination Act
1997	Faculty of Occupational Medicine's survey of members' occupational mental health experience and needs

(Miller, 1998). In many organisations it is occupational health departments which are leading the response to the psychological challenges of the workplace.

Statutory requirements and legal precedents have strengthened the case for intervention. The 1974 Health and Safety at Work Act established employers' responsibility for the health and safety of their employees. In 1992 the Management of Health and Safety at Work Regulations outlined more detailed responsibilities for employee health. However, organisations have been slow to develop consistent policies to protect the mental health of their staff.

The landmark case of *Walker* v. *Northumbria County Council* (see Chapter 4, Box 4.2, p. 30) proved to be a watershed in terms of employers' responses to the problems of stress at work. Walker, a senior social worker, obtained a judgement against his employers for breach of duty of care in failing to take reasonable steps to avoid exposing him to a health-endangering workload. The judgement emphasised that there was no reason why risk of psychiatric damage should be excluded from the scope of an employer's duty of care. Subsequent similar cases have resulted in substantial financial penalties.

The Disability Discrimination Act 1995 has provided a further stimulus to employers in this respect, as employees with a psychiatric condition recognised by a psychiatrist, or those who have a history of such a condition, are covered by it. The Act requires employers to consider the nature of the job in relation to the individual's ability and, where reasonably practicable, to modify the job requirements to enable an employee with a disability to work.

In addition to statutory requirements and legal precedents, the government has reaffirmed the need to address mental well-being in the workplace. One of the targets outlined in *Saving Lives: Our Healthier Nation* (Department of Health, 1999) was to 'Encourage employers to address stress at work'.

Developing an organisational strategy for mental health

The development of a successful organisational strategy for addressing mental health in the workplace starts with the adoption of a structured approach to measuring and managing the problem.

Employers are required to assess the risk to both the psychological and physical health of their employees. They have used various models to assess these risks, some of which include:

- the physical hazard model
- the general stress model

- the job demand/control model
- the vitamin model
- the affective events model (Briner, 2000).

The most commonly used are the general stress model and the physical hazard model. The general stress model is actually the basis of the physical hazards model. It proposes:

- a series of stressors on one side
- a series of effects on the other side
- modifying factors in between.

The physical hazard model, which was proposed by Griffiths & Cox (1996), mirrors one commonly used to identify physical hazards. This approach entails:

- identification of the hazard
- measurement of risk
- reduction of risk
- evaluation (audit).

Before proceeding with the identification of psychosocial hazards, it is important for the organisation to take ownership of the process through what might be labelled a 'development stage'.

Development stage

The support and energy of a champion at board level is critical at this stage. Different organisations will tailor the development process to suit their own structures, but one model would be to create a steering group. The terms of reference for this group might usefully include:

- identification of hazards to mental health
- development of risk assessment for these hazards
- development of procedures to reduce the risk to health
- development of evaluation procedures.

The steering group should be of workable size but might contain the following:

- a senior manager as chair
- a management representative
- a representative from occupational health
- a representative from safety
- representatives from the different disciplines within the organisation
- a representative from human resources
- staff/union representatives.

One of the first tasks of the group might be to agree a working title. Words such as 'stress' might not be acceptable and it might be better to look at alternative terms such as 'well-being', 'performance management' or 'lifestyle management'.

Identification of psychosocial hazards

At the assessment stage, the steering group will need to take an overall look at the organisation and gather information of various types, such as:

- general demographic and job information
- recognised psychosocial hazards within the organisation
- measured individual/group symptoms of stress
- measured outcomes (e.g. absenteeism, accidents, performance)
- existing interventions.

It is important to note that when identifying psychosocial hazards the group must look at aspects of the work environment that are relevant to workers' emotions, cognitions and behaviours.

The steering group may well be able to compile a list of the most obvious hazards to mental health in its particular organisation. It is often useful to develop a questionnaire tailored to the organisation which lists possible hazards. A good response to this (which can be encouraged by allowing respondents to be anonymous) will provide detailed information on employees' perceptions of stressors in their work environment and should help to prioritise interventions. It is usual to classify these hazards as organisational or job specific.

Organisational factors

There are six widely recognised organisational psychosocial hazards:

- organisational culture
- communications
- morale
- change
- inadequate personnel policies
- poor management.

Organisational culture

There are four broadly recognised organisational styles (Table 5.2). All have positive or negative effects on employee well-being.

Communications

A significant part of the structure of an organisation is the communication network. In practice it appears almost impossible to achieve adequate communication and in most organisations there is the

Table 5.2 The four organisational styles and their effects on employee well-being

Style	Characterisation
Power	The people in control use resources to control employees. This form of management is often known as 'Taylorism' or as 'stick and carrot management'. It is probably one of the most damaging and, although long since shown to be a poor form of management, is still present in many organisations.
Role	Everyone has clearly defined duties and rewards. The structure, routine and predictability provide security but are likely to restrict individuality and creativity. In the maelstrom of work today, many individuals yearn for such stability.
Achievement	Employees are lined up behind the organisation's mission statement. The personal energy of individuals is focused on the common goal. There is an expectation of total commitment that may be detrimental to family and social life. In such organisations you are only as good as your last 'whatever' (sales figures, budget management programme, etc.). In line with the thinking of management gurus, an increasing number of organisations are basing their working practices on this concept of employee identification with management aims.
Support	Based on mutual trust between the individual and the organisation, it is nurturing to most individuals, although dissatisfaction may be felt if equal reward is applied when there is not equal effort.

complaint that communication is poor both upwards and downwards. The perceived lack of downward communication becomes particularly critical at times of change and can be responsible for much stress and anxiety. However, communication overload also occurs. For example, the increasing use of email may be promoting a whole new area of psychological hazard because of the associated:

- increased workload
- opportunity for aggression
- opportunity for harassment
- substitution for face-to-face discussion/criticism
- opportunities for espionage.

Morale

Low morale is associated with high stress levels and if the organisation is not held in high regard publicly then employees are likely to become alienated from its aims. The belief that one is doing a worthwhile job in a worthwhile organisation can carry an individual healthily through pressured times (in the short term).

Change

It is difficult to think of any organisation that is not undergoing massive change. To most people change is associated with insecurity, either because of concomitant redundancies or because the job requirements are drastically changed and the individual may feel deskilled and vulnerable. Continuous change can stretch employees' adaptive and coping behaviours and so have an adverse effect on mental and physical well-being.

Inadequate personnel policies

As far as possible, employees need to know where they are in an organisation, and to feel that everyone will be treated fairly and with respect. Good personnel policies, which seek to safeguard these principles, should be in place and their absence may lead to much unnecessary anxiety.

Poor management

Another commonly perceived cause of stress is poor management. Individuals ascending the organisational ladder necessarily acquire an increased management role but frequently this is not accompanied by adequate management training. Indeed, particularly for those with specialist skills, the management part of their role may be regarded as an unimportant nuisance factor. The extent and effectiveness of management training are important factors in assessing risk to all areas of health.

Job-specific factors

Well-researched job-specific factors include:

- the nature of the work
- job overload
- interpersonal relationships
- job ambiguity and role conflict
- home–work conflicts.

The nature of the work

Although all work can be stressful, certain types of work are recognised as being more likely to induce stress:

- dealing with people and controlling groups of people
- monotonous work
- work with a risk of violence
- work involving short and unpredictable time-scales
- dirty work
- poorly regarded work
- work in hazardous situations
- work in exposed situations.

Job overload

One of the most common causes of stress at work is overload, where there is too much to do in too little time. Overload is compounded if the individual lacks control over inputs and if there are unrealistic deadlines. Overload can develop insidiously as tasks increase and, even if the individual perceives overload, it may not be possible to identify a solution without losing credibility or status.

Interpersonal relationships

If there is no relationship of mutual trust and respect between senior managers and other members of the team, the subordinate is likely to feel under pressure. Senior staff may feel equally under pressure when there is a mismatch between formal and actual power, or when a more democratic approach to decisions has been adopted. Unsatisfactory peer group relationships may cause more distress; 'scapegoating' is not unusual in work groups and cliques can develop.

Job ambiguity and role conflict

The lack of a clear or realistic job specification is a recognised risk factor which can lead to differing expectations between employee, manager and the peer group. Individuals may be responsible to more than one manager and have no clear guidance on priorities.

Home–work conflicts

Extended working hours and unsociable hours tend to disturb family and social life. Long hours of work may be the result of cultural imperatives rather than actual work demand.

The measurement of risk

Quantitative data in relation to risk assessment are often hard to find and this is particularly true for mental health hazards. A number of sources have, however, been used by various organisations and these include:

- human resources statistics
- stress audit
- questionnaire
- individual susceptibility.

Human resources statistics

Human resources departments maintain records on a wide variety of factors relating to the workforce. These statistics can help management quantify whether the organisation has a problem or not. The following statistics are particularly useful:

- sickness absence rates
- accident frequency
- staff turnover
- levels of temporary staff.

These statistics can be helpful in setting baselines and may often be a direct measure of the amount of stress within a department or organisation.

Stress audit

Various types of stress audits are available. Many of these are computer-based questionnaires that provide a means of identifying causes of stress and assessing coping abilities in individuals. They can also be used for group/department profiles identifying, for example, inter-personal or management problems. Such questionnaires are sensitive and many have normative data available, which allow findings to be compared with similar sector organisations. This type of comparison can be very helpful.

Questionnaire

Developing a questionnaire tailored to the organisation at the hazard identification stage will also give a clear indication of perceived risk.

Individual susceptibility

It is also important to look at the vulnerability of the individual and to recognise that there is a wide variation in individual resilience to pressure. Consequently, at the selection stage it is reasonable to consider whether the applicant's history or current psychological state suggests vulnerability to particular pressures. This is in line with current health and safety legislation, which requires the employer to consider individual susceptibility, and the Disability Discrimination Act 1995, which requires the employer to look at possible job modification. Both pieces of legislation also lay a duty on employers to monitor closely potential pressures following ill health.

Reducing the risk

Following hazard identification and risk assessment, the steering group will need to discuss the results and identify some of the key pressures within the organisation. These are likely to fall into three areas:

- *organisational* – interaction between employees and management, communication problems and organisational change
- *operational* – job specific
- *individual* – appraisal, career development, training.

Interventions may be either preventive (at the organisational or individual level) or supportive (of the employee). The steering group will need to decide at an early stage whether organisational engineering is appropriate or practical and whether individual intervention should be preventive or supportive.

Prevention – organisational

Changing the organisational culture

This requires commitment at the highest level and may be very difficult to achieve if the business style emanates from the most senior managers. Often cultures have developed over time and change can be incorporated into other business process re-engineering.

Improving the communication structure

The assessment of the communication structure should have included its effectiveness. Is communication really a two-way process so that information is exchanged or is it simply a cascading down of instructions? It may be necessary to examine the means of information dissemination and feedback processes.

Managing change

The modern age is an era of continuous change. It is therefore important that change is managed and that people are given skills not only to manage change but also to survive the change process. This may well be offered by workshops that provide information on the effects of change as well as individuals' personality to help them cope with change.

Improving management skills

The level of management training in the UK is generally below that of other European nations. There remains a misconception in many quarters that good management comes naturally. There are often particular difficulties with specialist staff moving into management and it is critical that everyone who is given management responsibility should also be provided with management training. The good manager should aim to be fair, understanding and reliable but should also not expect to be popular. A good manager also makes time to manage.

Developing health-related policies

The development of appropriate health-related policies can help both the individual and the organisation. Personnel policies that enshrine a caring response to mental ill health enable employees to reveal problems at an early stage, thus preventing the development of serious mental illness and long-term absence. Policies on sickness absence, disability, alcohol and other substance misuse, violence and harassment are particularly important and show that the organisation adopts a consistent approach to handling these issues. Also of benefit are socially sensitive initiatives such as flexitime, provision for working at home and crèche facilities, which reflect the increasing preponderance of women in many workforces. These may significantly decrease the stress experienced by staff, particularly women.

Managing rehabilitation

The rehabilitation of employees who have developed mental illness needs to be carefully managed and the penalties for not doing so have been highlighted by the Walker case. Guilt, stigma and a loss of self-confidence can be major barriers to a return to work and need to be carefully addressed. In some cases, mental illness may result in bizarre behaviour which is frightening to the observer and can sometimes be associated with danger; this may make it difficult for colleagues to accept the return to the workplace of someone who has just recovered from a mental illness.

Improving the person–environment fit

To improve the person–environment fit, changes may need to occur at a number of levels and procedures may need to be put in place to establish this commitment (see Table 5.3).

Prevention – individual

Stress management techniques/training

Training staff to manage pressure and cope with change is now commonplace. This type of training usually includes techniques for self-awareness, biofeedback, relaxation and exercise.

More recently, behavioural therapy techniques based on attribution have come into use with some success. The positioning of behaviour management training within general training programmes appears to be more acceptable and effective.

Health promotion packages

General health promotion can assist in the development of a sense of well-being and also give a message to staff that there is a caring management.

Table 5.3 Changes and procedures to improve the person–environment fit

Design	Management	Personnel
Job design	Culture	Selection
Work organisation	Management philosophy	Placement
Work procedures	Systems	Appraisal
Environment		Training

Employee support

Employee support programmes can be extensive and include:

- counselling/helplines
- medical screening and insurance
- exercise and relaxation
- group work (increasing social support).

It is important to provide a safe venue for staff for whom problems are developing and who may need some support and help to seek solutions.

Implementation

Once a decision on appropriate interventions has been made and agreed at the commissioning level, the steering group may need to continue to oversee implementation and set in place evaluation procedures.

Evaluation

To date, it has been difficult to assess the success of interventions to improve individual and organisational stress, as there is a dearth of information on the subject. Where there has been an attempt at evidence-based evaluation of interventions, the consistently best results have come from organisational changes. Enhanced employee support systems also seem to bring about improvement and to enhance employee satisfaction. Stress management training, on the other hand, has failed to show any consistent and sustained effect, and no intervention has been shown to be any better than any other. What is clear, however, is that the actual process of intervention (regardless of what the intervention is) seems to improve employee perceptions and attitudes and organisational culture. Repeating the pre-intervention question-naire is one common method of assessing the effect of changes, as are the less sensitive human resources statistics. Both methods can be compromised by other changes taking place in the business.

Conclusion

It has been argued that the methodology for the assessment of physical hazards is not appropriate to psychological hazards. The assessment of risk for physical hazards is relatively simple, because:

- physical hazards are context specific
- there is an identifiable dose–effect relationship
- their effects are always negative
- they are intrinsically harmful and only to a limited extent determined by individual susceptibility.

In addition, the nature of the harm caused by physical hazards is specific, whereas the harm caused by an adverse psychological environment may range from mild psychosomatic symptoms to psychiatric illness. However, as this system has the advantage of being familiar to managers and has achieved some sort of legitimacy, it remains a useful tool for the assessment of the psychological work environment.

There seems little doubt that, in the present climate of highly pressured work, organisations will need to demonstrate that they have in place an organisational plan to protect the mental health of their staff. The drivers for this are good management practice, health and safety law, and the risk of personal injury litigation. Most organisations have a long way to go in developing and implementing a structured approach to mental health. We have some building blocks and it is now time to begin to put them in place.

References

Briner, R. B. (2000) Relationships between work environments, psychological environments and psychological well-being. *Occupational Medicine*, **50**, 299–303.

Department of Health (1999) *Saving Lives: Our Healthier Nation*. London: Stationery Office.

Griffiths, A. & Cox, T. (1996) Employers' responsibilities for assessment and control of work-related stress: a European perspective. *Health and Hygiene*, **17**, 62–70.

Jones, J. R., Hodgson, J. T., Clegg, T. M., *et al* (1998) *Self-Reported Work-Related Illness in 1995. Results from a Household Survey*. London: Health and Safety Executive. http://www.hse.gov.uk/statistics/2002/swi95.pdf.

Miller, D. M. (1998) Improving mental well-being in the workplace. *Occupational Medicine*, **47**, 463–467.

Office of Population Censuses and Surveys (1992) *Labour Force Survey 1990 and 1991*. London: HMSO.

Smith, A. (2000) The scale of perceived occupational stress. *Occupational Medicine*, **50**, 294–298.

CHAPTER 6

Individual and organisational stress

Marian Roden and Stephen Williams

Definitions

'Stress' is a confusing and ambiguous term. It is used by managers and employees to describe a wide range of mental, physical and social ill health. To add to the confusion, stress is also used to describe a range of demands or pressures experienced by people at home and at work. The word 'stress' has been used to denote a stimulus *and* the response to that stimulus; a cause *and* the effect of that cause; it is even sometimes seen as a diagnosis on a medical certificate, although it is not a recognised medical condition. In consequence, the term needs clarifying and possibly redefining before it can be sensibly considered.

In the model we use, we distinguish between 'pressure' and 'stress'. Pressure is the starting point of the stress process, the stimulus in the stress equation. Pressure is inevitable and ubiquitous; it is neutral, being neither good nor bad; it is a component of 'challenge', without which we would never achieve our maximum potential. The distinction between pressure as an input and stress as an outcome shapes our definition of 'stress'. Stress is a negative imbalance in the system. Stress occurs when the perceived demands placed on the individual exceed that individual's ability to cope. In managing the stress process, we need to focus attention on each element: we need to look at the pressures on individual employees and at their ability to cope with that pressure in terms of their personality characteristics, particularly their locus of control and range of coping skills. Finally, we need to understand the interaction between pressure and coping in the causation of stress.

As Figure 6.1 shows, pressure can give rise to a positive or negative outcome, depending on how the individual perceives and responds to it. Our objective in managing individual and organisational stress is to improve the probability that pressure will produce a positive outcome – growth – rather than the negative outcome – stress.

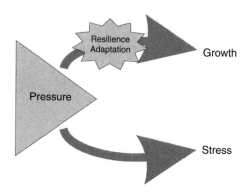

Figure 6.1 The relationship between pressure, growth and stress.

Causative factors

Pressures can derive from personal life as well as from work, the negative effects being indistinguishable and cumulative. In consequence, people who are experiencing stress in response to pressures at home, such as marital difficulties or problems with children, will come to work with a significant proportion of their coping capability already committed and therefore not available to accommodate workplace pressures. This provides companies with the rationale to help employees cope with pressure generally, and not just with pressure at work, since the two are inextricably linked.

A list of all possible workplace pressures would be virtually endless; Table 6.1 attempts to capture the most common and important workplace stressors.

Table 6.1 The most common and important workplace stressors

Source of pressure	Description
Workload	The amount or difficulty of your work
Relationships	How well you get on with the people you work with
Recognition	The extent to which you feel that your efforts and achievements are recognised
Organisational climate	The 'feel' or 'atmosphere' within your place of work
Personal responsibility	Being responsible for your actions and decisions
Managerial role	Being responsible for managing and supervising others
Home–work balance	'Switching off' from the pressure of work when at home, and vice versa
Daily hassles	The day-to-day irritants and aggravations in the workplace

Clinical presentation

The manifestations of stress are many and varied, and stress has been cited as causing and/or aggravating a large number of medical conditions. The symptoms and signs of stress can be classified as physical, psychological and behavioural. A number of the more common ones are listed below; although these can all be caused by stress, they can also occur in other circumstances.

Physical

The physical presentations of stress include:

- altered sleep patterns, such as difficulty getting to sleep, early waking
- tiredness
- lethargy
- panic attacks – breathlessness, bouts of dizziness, light-headedness
- dyspeptic symptoms
- nausea
- bowel symptoms, such as diarrhoea, constipation
- headaches
- muscle tension, such as neck pain, back pain
- nervous twitches.

Psychological

The psychological presentations of stress include:

- irritability and aggression
- anxiety and depression
- poor decision-making
- preoccupation with trivia
- inability to prioritise
- difficulty in coping
- mood changes and swings
- difficulty in concentrating
- deterioration in recent memory
- feelings of failure
- lack of self-worth.

Behavioural

The behavioural presentations of stress include:

- lack of concern for appearance
- altered eating habits – more or less appetite
- drinking more

- smoking more
- absenteeism
- more accidents
- 'presenteeism' – being physically at work, but not performing satisfactorily.

Prognosis

The prognosis is generally good, provided the root causes are identified and successfully tackled. However, as with all illness, early detection and prompt treatment will improve the chances of a positive outcome.

Effect on work

Stress can have a negative effect on practically all aspects of performance, as can the drugs used to treat anxiety and depression. Particular consideration should be given to those driving or operating machinery; those in jobs where accuracy is critical; and those whose decisions have significant impact on the organisation.

Interventions

Interventions are traditionally divided into primary, secondary and tertiary. Primary interventions seek to remove or modify the cause at source; secondary interventions seek to equip people to deal more effectively with the pressures they encounter in life; tertiary interventions seek to treat damage already done. The underlying model of stress emphasises the need to understand the sources of pressure and, as a consequence, focuses attention on primary interventions. However, because of the multifactorial nature of occupational stress, many organisations find it difficult to deal with the source of the problem and, instead, focus their attention on the visible outcome of the stress process, that is, those individuals who are suffering from stress-related illnesses. We therefore have a situation in many organisations where efforts to reduce workplace stress are misplaced, and interventions are concentrated at the remedial (tertiary) level, not the primary level. Stress is then wrongly perceived as the problem of the individual and not of the organisation, whereas, in fact, like most health and safety issues, it is best seen as a shared responsibility.

Primary interventions

The Health and Safety Executive (1995) takes the view that psychological pressure at work must be approached in the same way as any other workplace hazard. It must be assessed and where found to be excessive, appropriately modified. The use of questionnaires such as the Pressure Management Indicator (Williams & Cooper, 1996) provides a structure for the analysis of the nature and extent of occupational stress and helps the design of interventions that meet the specific needs of the organisation. Relying exclusively on secondary and tertiary interventions is no more acceptable in the area of pressure than it is in the area of noise, where we are required to reduce noise at source before we resort to handing out ear defenders and hearing aids.

Some examples of primary interventions are improving job design, enhancing management skills, modifying organisational culture, introducing flexible systems of work and enhancing leadership skills.

Secondary interventions

Although primary interventions must never be overlooked, there is a place for secondary interventions as well. Because pressure is inevitable and because much of it arises outside the workplace and is therefore beyond the control of occupational physicians, it makes sense to teach people the skills to manage pressure effectively and positively. We have already established that work affects home and vice versa; therefore, if we can help people to manage pressure more effectively, then we can expect a resultant improvement in their ability to perform.

There are many types of 'stress management' course, from those that concentrate on the three 'C's of control, challenge and commitment to those that take the wider view that pressure management is a subset of self-management, and that if you manage yourself effectively then stress ceases to be an issue. Stress management also draws from the areas of assertiveness training and time management. Our experience shows that understanding the dynamics of the stress process should be a core component of any 'pressure management' training. Many people have little understanding of the physiological component of the stress reaction. Explaining the physiology of the fight-or-flight reaction helps employees to recognise that the way they feel is a function of an inappropriate evolutionary response. This understanding removes the 'fear' of stress and overcomes the common feeling that admitting to stress is a sign of weakness and individual failure.

A very effective approach to pressure management is the concept of building resilience at both the individual and organisational level. If we concentrate on the individual without attending to the organisation, we are simply cleaning up the fish only to put it back in the dirty pond. The most successful approach is a two-pronged one in which we teach individuals the behaviours and competencies of personal resilience, while working on cultural issues and leadership competencies to improve the organisational environment. An example here is the issue of work–life balance. A characteristic of resilient people is that they consistently display the ability to balance their work and personal lives in a manner which is satisfactory to them; the organisation can support this behaviour by implementing flexible systems of work, supporting diversity and stamping out any long-hours culture.

Tertiary interventions

In the noise reduction analogy, these are the hearing aids. Examples are employee assistance programmes and counselling services. While these are in no way a satisfactory response to the stress issue on their own, they do provide the comfort of a safety net. They also cater for those whose primary stressors lie in their personal lives and are therefore beyond the company's control, but the company can expect a payback in the form of a more speedily rehabilitated employee. The danger in an over-reliance on counselling is that organisations believe they have 'dealt with' stress, when in fact they have failed to move beyond the outward signs to get at the root causes.

Despite an enormous amount of work and numerous information campaigns, there is, in many organisations, still a stigma attached to mental health in general and stress in particular. Introducing the issue of stress under the banner of pressure management makes the subject more acceptable to employers and encourages employees to participate in programmes without admitting that they can no longer cope.

References

Health and Safety Executive (1995) *Stress at Work*. London: HSE.
Williams, S. & Cooper, C. L. (1996) *The Pressure Management Indicator*. Harrogate: RAD Ltd.

Further reading

Cooper, C. L. & Williams, S. (eds) (1994) *Creating Healthy Work Organisations*. Chichester: John Wiley & Sons.
Covey, S. (1989) *The Seven Habits of Highly Effective People*. London: Simon & Schuster.
Williams, S. (1994) *Managing Pressure for Peak Performance*. London: Kogan Page.

CHAPTER 7

A team approach to managing mental health at work: the AstraZeneca case study

Richard Heron

Background

Life in the modern world presents great challenges to both people and organisations. The ability to balance often competing demands from the workplace and the home is a skill that needs to be developed. Success leads to well motivated and well-rounded people who are capable of giving of their best in all aspects of their lives. AstraZeneca employs over 50 000 staff, of whom 11 000 are based in the UK. The company operates globally in the increasingly competitive pharmaceuticals market, with ever more rigorous demands from regulatory authorities. This is a challenging working environment and the company recognises the importance of keeping staff motivated, as well as maintaining their health and well-being.

A model for mental well-being

AstraZeneca's model of well-being has been developed and refined over recent years. It is based on a variety of different ideas, which have been adopted and tailored to meet the needs of the company. The model describes a continuum of mental well-being, ranging from serious health problems to personal fulfilment, and highlights the areas where companies can support individuals not only for their own benefit but for that of the business.

The interventions employed to promote well-being and reduce mental illness and its effects are many and varied. They range from normal good management practice, such as matching skills to jobs, training and development, through to the recognition and management of mental illness in a workplace setting. The model recognises that at any time the mental health status of members of the workforce is likely to span the (few) seriously impaired to the highly fulfilled. Staff who are unwell are less likely to perform to a high standard and contribute to the success of the company than those who are healthy. The focus is therefore on creating and sustaining an environment which supports development and fulfilment so that the well-being of staff is realised through policies and practices which centre on managers organising work appropriately. In this way the mental well-being of the company as a whole can be ensured.

Successful application of the model requires the senior management team to be committed to an organisational framework and management practices which support these aims. Within AstraZeneca, the Chief Executive and the Senior Executive Team (SET) have visibly and actively recognised these aims. Examples of this have included senior management stating to all employees that they recognise the pressures they experience, targeting workplace pressure management as a key area for improvement, and including the subject of work–life balance as a topic for discussion at a meeting of the top 150 senior managers. In addition to these initiatives, the Chief Executive's Award for Safety, Health and Environment (in 2001) rewarded the best submission for excellence in the area of 'Health and Well-being'.

Occupational health professionals have worked with the SET to update them regularly on mental health issues within the organisation, while protecting individual confidentiality. This has enabled them to ensure that appropriate policies are in place and that suitable training is provided to support staff.

Policies and guidelines

The company's safety, health and environment (SHE) policy covers all elements of its activities, including the health and well-being of employees. Under the umbrella of this broad policy, eight standards have been set which are mandatory and set the requirements to secure implementation of the policy. The company has produced guidelines which are designed to help managers comply with the standards and apply good practice.

One of the guidelines is targeted at maintaining and improving mental well-being at work. The focus is on the use of primary preventive strategies and the adoption of good management practices, such as open communications, appropriate job design, appropriate work scheduling, skills training, adequate resourcing and appropriate reward. Other areas in which good practice is encouraged are health promotion and rehabilitation.

Training is provided to help managers minimise the adverse impact of stress and to promote a supportive environment which encourages a healthy lifestyle. It also seeks to encourage those with stress-related problems to seek help. Stress and pressure management training workshops provide information on stress, signs of stress and stress management, and raise the topics of relaxation and time management. They may flag up, for some individuals, the need for training in such things as assertiveness, delegation, coaching, project management skills or negotiation skills. Such training is targeted to meet the needs of specific groups. Training sessions available include pressure management workshops for senior managers, and managers of teams, and coping skills for non-managers.

An integrated approach

A key strategic objective for the business, within the broad well-being philosophy, is to achieve a well motivated workforce who experience job satisfaction, and a focus on managing work within the overall life context. The emphasis is on an integrated approach to helping people develop themselves and their capabilities, not only for work but also in all other aspects of their lives.

In order to determine what actions should be taken to improve personal well-being for the benefit of the individual and business, AstraZeneca held meetings with a wide range of staff, including national site managers, occupational health specialists, human resource professionals, safety managers and infrastructure managers. Similar groups met in other countries where AstraZeneca operates to identify shared principles which could be interpreted in a locally and culturally appropriate way.

It is important to ensure that the needs of those who have a role to play in promoting employee well-being are also met. The company has therefore set up a leadership programme which is attended by senior managers. The programme provides an opportunity for these managers to reflect on key issues affecting personal and business performance, and issues of work–life balance and managing pressure effectively are frequent topics of discussion.

The CALM programme

Access to confidential counselling has been an important part of the overall strategy. In the early 1990s, counselling was provided by an industrial chaplain and an occupational health nurse. In 1996 the company, then Zeneca, established the CALM (Counselling And Life Management) programme. The programme is now jointly sponsored by the occupational health and the human resources functions. Following the merger with Astra, the CALM programme was extended nationally with on-site counselling provided at the larger sites and overseen by local steering groups inclusive of human resources, health and employee representatives.

The CALM programme has a code of ethics and a code of practice. It is designed to help people achieve and maintain balanced lives. It is run as a confidential service and it provides the opportunity for individuals to work towards living in a more satisfying and resourceful way. It aims to help them to make their own choices and decisions and to put them into action. All employees receive details about CALM.

The role of the CALM team is not limited to the provision of individual support. Information for managers is generated by recording the areas of concern which lead to counselling appointments, although the identity of individuals is strictly protected. This has facilitated further targeted and integrated support for the workforce, which may focus on specifics, such as business policies on bullying and harassment, for example, or may lead to a health-based response. CALM encourages the consideration of life management so that people can better recognise the signs of stress, explore their own personal strengths and weaknesses, and develop coping mechanisms. It provides them with options for support. CALM counselling is entirely voluntary, even if an individual has been referred by management. It is well used. CALM also links with external resources, such as the Citizens' Advice Bureau and specialist counselling services.

Staff consult the CALM team for a wide variety of reasons (Figure 7.1). Analysis of data arising from the programme not only provides feedback to help direct management action but also provides a focus for

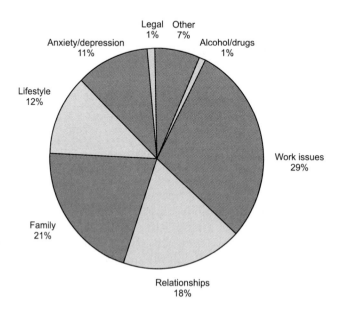

Figure 7.1 Reasons for staff consulting the Counselling And Life Management (CALM) team.

initiatives, such as training, presentations and self-help leaflets aimed at improving mental well-being.

The CALM team strives to make sure that the programme remains responsive to the needs of employees and management. Local steering committees comprise a senior management representative (often the site manager), an occupational health professional, a human resources manager, the CALM team of counsellors and employee representatives (often a union representative) from different levels on major sites. The steering groups ensure the cultural sensitivity of the service and obtain general feedback from employees about current issues. The CALM team regularly updates the steering group, employee representatives and senior managers regarding the issues raised by contact through the programme, although individual confidentiality is scrupulously maintained.

Counselling services are a key element in the organisational philosophy of 'well-being', but other activities also contribute. These include a comprehensive programme of training by occupational health professionals and a variety of health education initiatives. Staff also have access to fitness facilities as well as various activities available through a leisure club, together with a health promotion programme offering advice on a variety of topics. Training, health promotion and CALM initiatives all provide support to staff in need. The ready availability of professional occupational health staff has proved critical to those in crisis and has facilitated prompt referral to the employee's medical practitioner or specialist where appropriate.

Evaluation of interventions

It is considered vital to monitor the extent of interventions together with the effect that they have had. As a consequence, data on the uptake of counselling, the use of health centres and the monitoring of training activities are collected. Evaluation is carried out by the use of well-researched instruments, which provide an assessment of mental well-being over time. These include the General Health Questionnaire (GHQ; Goldberg, 1972) and elements of the Occupational Stress Indicator (OSI; Copper et al, 1988), as well as others covering life events and coping skills. Research suggests that attending the stress management training workshops is associated with a short-term improvement in well-being, as well as a greater understanding of the principles of stress management (Heron et al, 1999). The results of these evaluations are widely shared with management and staff at all levels within the company.

There are a number of other mechanisms which are used within the business to assess employees' sense of well-being and to identify areas for potential focus. The use of employee surveys is a well-recognised technique to allow staff to register their views and, occasionally, concerns. By working closely with the human resources department, a 'well-being' index of questions has been incorporated within the employee survey. This provides managers with a tool to identify 'hot-spots' and significant organisational issues associated with suboptimal well-being (e.g. workload, home–work interface, flexible working practices, opportunities for development and management support). Local human resources, occupational health and CALM staff are then able to provide assistance in progressing positive actions to address them.

Training surveys, such as those conducted for the 'Investors in People' process, and auditing provide additional data, which are used to help assess the general well-being of employees and identify where improvements might be made.

Mental well-being central to business success

Mental illness itself is common in the working-age population. A survey by the Office of Population, Census and Surveys (1994) has confirmed that one in seven adults (aged 16–64 years) living in private households were suffering from a mental health problem, such as anxiety or depression, in the week before interview (Meltzer *et al*, 1994). The scale of the problem makes it inevitable that almost all employees and businesses will confront mental illness at some time. Making sure that mental health problems are recognised at an early stage and offering access to confidential support in a workplace setting therefore makes sense for both the individual and the employer.

Management of pressure at AstraZeneca is now much more than an organisational add-on to occupational health services. It is an integral part of managing the business. Managers regularly seek advice about organisational changes proposed, so that mental distress can be minimised, and occupational health staff are routinely invited to comment on new working arrangements. Stress and pressure manage-ment programmes and access points to the counselling service are integrated within departmental training portfolios and information sources. Pressures affecting staff can never be removed – this is a normal part of life. We all now live in an ever-changing, complex global operating environment. However, by close cooperation between occu-pational health staff, human resources, management at all levels and all employee groups it has been possible to identify, prioritise and take actions to improve life management issues to the benefit of all in the company.

Conclusion

AstraZeneca recognises the need to maintain and enhance the health of its staff. The main focus is on encouraging management practices that maintain health and raise the self-esteem of staff. This approach is supplemented by training in specific tasks and 'life skills'. Having ready access to confidential support and access to specialist skills is also valuable.

Good health should lead to a happy, productive workforce. This is one of the fundamentals of ensuring a good and profitable business.

References

Cooper C. L., Sloan, S. J. & Williams, S. (1988) *Occupational Stress Indicator*. Windsor: NFER.

Goldberg, D. (1972) *The Detection of Psychiatric Illness by Questionnaire*. Oxford: Oxford University Press.

Heron, R. J. L., McKeown, S., Tomenson, J. & Teasdale, E. L. (1999) Study to evaluate the effectiveness of stress management workshops on response to general and occupational measures of stress. *Occupational Medicine*, **49**, 451–457.

Meltzer, H., Gill, B. & Pettigrew, M. (1994) The prevalence of psychiatric morbidity among adults aged 16–64, living in private households in Great Britain. *OPCS Surveys of Psychiatric Morbidity in Great Britain*, bulletin no. 1.

CHAPTER 8

Managing pressure:
the Marks & Spencer case study

Noel McElearney

The background

Marks & Spencer, one of the UK's leading retailers, is known as a caring employer that invests substantial resources into its personnel activities. One of the organisation's key principles is 'Care of the Individual' and it is in this area that occupational health makes a significant contribution. Marks & Spencer's staff typically give long service to the business and develop long-term relationships with suppliers. However, retailing is a business in which detail is important. There is constant change, driven by seasonal and competitive factors. At Marks & Spencer the focus is always on improving the 5% that did not go well. Standards and expectations are high. Stretched targets are normal.

It is against this background that the occupational health department first recognised the need to work on stress management. However, when designing a programme the department had to be sensitive to the fact that this way of working (high standards, stretched targets, etc.) is common in customer-led businesses, and retailing in particular.

None of this is new and indeed mental ill health was first recognised as a problem in retailers by Charles Turner Thackrah, in his book *The Effects of Arts, Trades and Professions on Health and Longevity*, published in 1831. He said:

'Shopkeepers are pale, dyspeptic and subject to affections of the head. They often drag on a sickly existence, die before the proper end of human life and leave a progeny like themselves.'

He went on to note that:

'Anxiety of the mind does more I conceive to impair health. The body suffers from the mind, that sense of responsibility which every conscientious practitioner must feel – the anxious zeal that makes him throw his mind and feelings into cases of especial danger, break down the frame, change the face of hilarity to that of seriousness and care and bring on premature age.'

Thackrah's description of work-related mental ill health remains as relevant today as when first published. It even captures the fact that the best employees – the conscientious practitioners – may be the very ones at risk and that these employees may become ill when the business can least afford it.

The agenda

Like many big organisations, Marks & Spencer has a unique culture. Years of experience have led people to establish a set way of working. One example is the use of consultation. In Marks & Spencer there is a need to consult widely before proceeding with any initiative. Indeed, if you do not consult beforehand your idea may meet with rejection.

Marks & Spencer is also an empirical business. It tests and evaluates, it carries out trials of its goods and its services; it has model stores and gauges customer reaction regularly. It commits itself to a 'measure it to manage it' way of work.

Bearing this in mind, the occupational health department believed that the only way in which to get stress on the agenda – in a way that would meet with acceptance – would be by consulting extensively and by adopting an empirical approach. However, in order to provide valid empirical measurements, the department needed a tool that would provide a reliable measure of stress and that could be understood by every level of user.

The department elected to use the Organisational Stress Indicator (OSI), which has now been superseded by the Pressure Management Indicator (PMI). The PMI was selected on the basis that it had been extensively validated and allowed comparison with other working populations, and because the occupational health department believed that it utilised a model of stress that would work well in the retail business.

The PMI

The psychological model upon which the PMI is based (Figure 8.1) is dynamic. In this model, sources of pressure are counterbalanced by an individual's skills to cope with it. Personality strongly influences the outcome. These factors shift to create either positive or negative outcomes.

In order to measure the individual's level of stress, the PMI probes the following:

- sources of pressure
- factors influencing ability to cope
- coping mechanisms and effects.

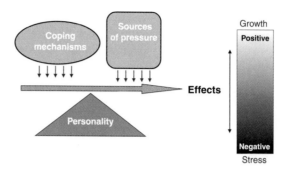

Figure 8.1 The dynamics of the stress process. (Source: Dr Stephen Williams, Resources Systems, Harrogate, UK. With permission.)

Each of these areas is examined by asking groups of related questions. This generates a series of sub-scales. Table 8.1 shows the items measured by each of these. Like all questionnaires, there are internal validating questions. A total of 120 questions are asked and, on average, it takes about 20 minutes to complete.

Once an individual has completed the PMI, the questionnaire is scored and the individual is provided with the results. These results include information on how the individual compares with the general working population. The report provides an excellent starting point for discussion on the subject of work-related stress. It should, however, never be considered as a substitute for discussing the report with a facilitator who is trained to interpret the results.

The Marks & Spencer case

Marks & Spencer has an extensive nationwide occupational health presence that keeps its finger on the pulse of the organisation. Based on its knowledge of the organisation, the occupational health department believed that it needed to develop a programme that would meet the needs of the majority of staff – namely, those who are well but interested in the subject of stress – and not the minority who might be stressed. This decision was made on the basis that the department could deal with individual cases internally once overall awareness of the issue had been raised. The next stage was to determine the strategic objectives and design of the initiative.

The occupational health department knew from extensive bench-marking with staff that they valued personal contact. Consequently, it would not be enough to have staff only complete a questionnaire: some form of facilitated intervention was required. Additionally, when designing any intervention, the department had to bear in mind the

Table 8.1 The PMI sub-scales

Contents of the scale	Nature of question
Satisfaction	
Job satisfaction	Your satisfaction with the type of work you do
Organisation satisfaction	Your satisfaction with the way your organisation is structured and the way it works
The organisation	
Organisational security	How you feel about the stability of your organisation and your level of job security
Organisational commitment	How committed you are to the organisation and the extent to which you enjoy your job, and feel that work improves the quality of your life
Mental well-being	
State of mind	Your level of mental well-being
Resilience	Your ability to 'bounce back' from setbacks or problems
Confidence level	How worried you are
Physical well-being	
Physical symptoms	How calm you feel in terms of physical tension or other uncomfortable sensations
Energy	The amount of energy and vitality you have
Sources of pressure	
Workload	The amount or difficulty of work you have to deal with
Relationships	How well you get on with those around you, particularly those at work
Recognition	The extent to which you feel you need to have your achievements recognised
Organisational climate	The 'feel' or 'atmosphere' within your place of work
Personal responsibility	Taking responsibility for your actions and decisions
Managerial role	Taking responsibility for managing and supervising other people
Home–work balance	'Switching off' from the pressure of work when at home, and vice versa
Daily hassles	The day-to-day irritants and aggravations in the workplace
Behaviour	
Drive	Your desire to succeed and achieve results
Patience/impatience	Your pace of life and your ability to cope with your need for urgency
Control/influence	
Control	The extent to which you feel able to influence and control events
Personal influence	How much influence you have over your work and are able to exercise discretion in your job
Coping	
Problem focus	The extent to which you feel able to plan ahead and manage your time to deal with problems
Emotional detachment	The extent to which you are able to separate home from work and not let things get to you
Support	
Social support	The help you get by discussing problems or situations with other people

Source: Dr Stephen Williams, Resources Systems, Harrogate, UK. With permission.

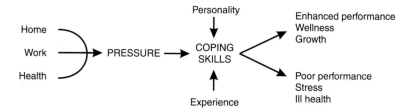

Figure 8.2 Different sources of pressure combine to interact with personality and experience, in the form of coping skills, to produce a range of effects, from good to bad.

demographics of the organisation, as this would affect the needs of the workforce. At Marks & Spencer the workforce is 85% female and mostly part time. The programme therefore had to take into account the effect of what was happening at the employee's home, as it is known that non-work pressure contributes significantly to the total pressure employees face (Figure 8.2)

In view of the above factors, the department set the following strategic objectives:

- choose a definition of stress and 'stick to it'
- raise awareness of the issue at all levels in the business
- heighten awareness of the impact of home life and personal health
- clarify the fact that the solutions are managerial and not medical
- establish that working under pressure in the long term requires additional skills.

These objectives were to be met by holding workshops and asking staff to complete the PMI questionnaire.

Trial workshops

The first trial was a conventional two-day workshop. It included everything anyone could ever hope to know about stress. It was medically oriented and it had a lot of material on adrenaline, fear, fight and flight. It explained how employees could recognise the signs and symptoms of stress in themselves and in others. It also covered coping strategies, relaxation, diet and exercise. Employees were provided with a workbook, course materials and a PMI questionnaire. The staff called it 'comprehensive'.

The second trial consisted of 12 one-day workshops co-presented by a personnel manager and an occupational health adviser. On this occasion, the content focused more on health rather than the medical consequences of stress. Employees continued to receive the PMI questionnaire; however, they were also provided with a pre-course workbook. Unfortunately, as is often the case, the delegates did not do their homework before attending the course. They did, however, use the workbook as a reference after they completed the workshop.

The feedback on the workbook was so positive that a decision was made to publish its content as a booklet. The end result was a booklet entitled *Manage Your Pressure*. To date, the organisation has distributed about 25 000 copies. Staff have found it very useful and are particularly happy to see pictures of men being stressed!

With regard to the trial of the second workshop itself, staff told us that they were happy to have occupational health advisers deliver the course but that the personnel managers 'somehow got in the way'. Much of this response was related to the fact that the advisers were perceived as neutral and well informed.

In the third trial the course was pared down to a half-day workshop presented solely by an occupational health adviser. Once again, staff received the PMI questionnaire and this time materials were distributed during the course. The participants were also provided with information about further sources of help within health services. The feedback on the third trial was very favourable and as a result the department of occupational health believed that it had found a format that would meet all of its original objectives.

Staff workshops – current experience

Since the development of the course, about 800 delegates (in groups of 12) have participated in the programme and nearly 20 of the organisation's occupational health advisers have been trained as facilitators.

The organisation targets any group that might benefit from examining the issue of stress, and experience has shown that it is best to keep people from similar jobs together, as this often promotes the development of shared solutions. For example, sales assistants and supervisors have limited power to create change but they do have enough to make a significant impact on their own stores. It is not really surprising how expert people can be in finding solutions to their own problems. In fact, when this is done in a group setting, people are more likely to try it and to sustain the changes.

Developing a management training programme

Throughout the course of the workshops, sales assistants and supervisors consistently told us that, relatively speaking, they were fine, but that we ought to see the managers! Marks & Spencer managers are surely the retailers that Thackrah had in mind. They are conscientious practitioners. They measure it and manage it. They move it and measure it again. Retailing is both a science and an art. In general, it seems that Marks & Spencer managers in each other's company will talk about yield, knickers and bananas, football, footfall and profitability. It is a 'macho' world so there is not much room for 'touchy feely' stuff. But as we move closer and closer to 24-hour operations and 365-day-a-year trading, they, too, are beginning to realise the need for balance in their lives. Whereas in the beginning stress was fine for the general staff, managers now ask 'What about us?'

Many stress courses are didactic. They identify problem lists that are similar for most organisations, and that include, for example, too much work, not enough staff, loss of home–work partitions, and job insecurity. Each one of these is amenable to well-known management solutions. So why does the problem persist?

The occupational health department believes that two issues contribute to this: first, the inability to recognise stress; and second, the imposition of inappropriate solutions. The Marks & Spencer management workshops have therefore been designed to overcome these problems. Thus the workshops focus on helping managers recognise stress. Being stressed is a lot like suffering from hypertension – you may not know you have it until some event occurs. Building awareness is therefore a key preventive strategy. The message also has to be delivered in a way that does not threaten self-esteem.

In addition to helping managers recognise stress, the workshop is being used as a forum to launch new management ideas that take into account the changing nature of the organisation, and help managers understand and develop the skills they will need to move forward with the organisation. For example, at Marks & Spencer there has been a shift away from old-fashioned styles of management: there is now much more emphasis on team skills. The organisation has empowered supervisors and sales assistants and devolved decision-making to lower levels. However, you cannot lead those teams without some sensitivity to interpersonal skills. The ability to partition (home–work balance) and to bounce back from disappointment has also become increasingly important.

Just as it is critical to approach the diagnosis carefully, and to introduce managers to new management ideas, it is equally important to recognise that fixing the problem is something people can do only for themselves. A thousand management texts can tell you what to do, but only the individual and the group know how to fit that solution into their unique context. It is just as important for managers to come to that realisation. The new managers' course, which Marks & Spencer is developing by a trial process, embraces all of these principles. As well as launching new management ideas, the workshop format contains ideas borrowed from solution-focused therapy, thereby moving away from the concept of 'imposed solutions'.

Managing Pressure for Managers – the course

Managing Pressure for Managers is a day and a half long, residential and held well away from the workplace. Internal and external tutors lead the course.

On the first afternoon delegates are introduced to the issues related to individual and organisational stress. It is made clear that it must be managed. Tutors explain how humans have improperly evolved physiologically for their current roles and that, therefore, stress occurs because individuals are human, not because they are weak. The course then links how psychological threats can produce similar physiological responses as physical threats.

Early the next morning everyone goes for a run. This has the benefit of linking a physical experience to the physiology as taught the preceding evening. It reinforces that what is happening is true. It has the other benefit of eliminating any remaining adrenaline. Participants are more relaxed for the remainder of the day.

Much of the morning is devoted to problem-solving techniques (borrowed heavily from solution-focused therapy). The managers practise these techniques in small groups using issues that are common to them all. This enables them not only to learn how to use these techniques but also to find solutions that they can use when they return to work. Since these techniques can be applied in any setting, they can also use these skills to resolve non-work-related problems.

Conclusion

The course not only met the set objectives but it was also well received by the delegates. It has created sustained change, as shown by the fact that the changes in lifestyle and interpersonal relations that were stimulated by the pilot courses have been sustained over a year for many of the individuals who took part.

CHAPTER 9

Supporting mental well-being through the promotion of a balanced lifestyle

Marian Roden

The characteristics of resilience

Mental well-being is a characteristic of resilient people – the sort of people who not only survive but thrive in situations of high pressure and challenge. These are people who are able to say 'Whatever life throws at me, I know I will be able to cope' and believe it. Such people demonstrate adaptability and flexibility in fast-paced, pressured and culturally diverse environments; they display confidence, energy and stamina in meeting challenging goals; and they draw on other areas of life to maintain a healthy and balanced perspective.

The basic attributes of resilient people (adapted from Conner, 1995) are that they are:

- positive – they display self-assurance and a sense of security
- focused – they have a clear vision of what they want to achieve
- flexible – they demonstrate pliability when faced with uncertainty
- organised – they develop structured approaches to managing ambiguity
- proactive – they engage change rather than defending against it
- energetic – they display high levels of physical, emotional and intellectual energy.

Resilient people are also characterised by a number of behaviours, beliefs and attitudes, all of which can be learned and practised by those who wish to enhance their personal resilience. These 'building blocks' of resilience are:

- life balance
- effective pressure management
- self-responsibility
- identification of personal values and a sense of purpose in life
- prioritisation and time management
- effective decision-making
- flexible or learned optimism (Seligman, 1992)
- continuous personal renewal and self-development.

Life balance

The first of these 'building blocks' of resilience is a balanced lifestyle. Resilient people consistently display the ability to balance and integrate the various aspects of their lives in a way that is satisfactory for them. Balance means different things to different people, because it is based on personal values and there is consequently no universally applicable standard. All individuals have different values and will choose to integrate the various aspects of their lives in different ways, in accordance with those values. The balance will alter at different points in a person's life. For example, a young man might consciously choose to spend a lot of time and energy on his career, when he is fresh out of college, single and starting a new job; he will want to establish a firm foothold on his career ladder. However, ten years later, when he is married and has a newborn child at home, what he values and how he chooses to integrate the various aspects of his life might change significantly. If he, his wife or child develops a life-threatening illness, his values might change again. Essentially, the right balance varies between individuals and for each individual at different stages in life.

It is unrealistic to seek to achieve a constant steady state of perfect balance; a more practical aspiration is for a flexible, responsive balance. Stephen Covey describes this goal as 'a lifetime of balance with seasons of imbalance' (Covey et al, 1995). Individuals may well choose for a time to focus on one aspect of life at the expense of the others. This is unlikely to cause psychological harm provided that it is for a limited period and that thereafter the balance is redressed. Problems occur when long periods of imbalance result and the individual rationalises the situation as being just temporary. Most people can maintain an imbalance for a short period, but if it persists it is likely to lead not only to damage to the neglected areas but also, eventually, to a breakdown of overall health and well-being.

An analogy for this is to imagine a tree in which the roots represent key areas in a person's life. A feature of healthy trees is that the spread of their roots is almost as wide as the height of the tree. This gives the tree mechanical stability and enables it to draw its nutrients from a wide area of soil. If one of the roots hits a rock, is temporarily damaged or enters a patch of poisoned soil, the others will keep the tree alive. If an adverse life event occurs – a strong gust of wind in this analogy – the tree's inherent stability will keep it upright and enable it to survive.

However, if that same tree had a single tap root, it would be less able to withstand adversity. Such examples are rare in nature, but this is precisely what occurs in people's lives when they persistently neglect some of their fundamental needs. No matter how thick, long and well developed this single root is, if it is damaged or enters a patch of bad soil, the tree will die. Similarly, it is obvious that this tree is inherently unstable, so that a strong wind (in our analogy an adverse life event, such as the loss of a job or the death of a loved one) may knock it down, snap its sole root and it will die.

As stated earlier, energy is an attribute of resilience. Energy is enhanced by good health, which is itself a component of resilience. Enhanced health and energy can be achieved by focusing on our basic needs – physical, intellectual, social, emotional and spiritual. These needs may be acknowledged, denied or ignored but unless they are attended to, health and productivity will, in due course, be impaired.

Compartmentalisation *v.* integration

One of the reasons many people find it difficult to keep their lives in balance is that they have a 'compartmentalised' view of life. They see the different key areas of their lives as competing against, rather than supporting, each other, and the only way they can give attention to one is by taking away from another. The different areas of their lives are thus perceived as being in conflict. The result is that they try to live their lives like a baseball game, attempting to run faster and faster so that they touch each base at least once every day. This approach is doomed to failure since it inevitably leads to energy depletion and exhaustion.

By contrast, an 'integrated' view of life sees the different dimensions as supporting one another. When an individual attends to one area of life, other dimensions are automatically enhanced at the same time. In this model, the different areas are no longer in conflict. For example, if one goes out and exercises – maybe takes a brisk walk – one not only feels physically better for it but one also feels psychologically better. When we feel psychologically better, our mental powers become sharper and, as a result, we become more creative, we make better decisions, our memory improves and we think and process information more efficiently and effectively. Moreover, when we feel psychologically good, our relationships go well, and this improves our social and emotional life. That is how the integrated model works. When the dimensions of people's lives are all attended to and they are balanced, it is then that they will find that they are happy, healthy and productive and able to perform to the best of their abilities.

This is particularly pertinent to the balance between work and personal life. If a person sees work and personal life from a compartmentalised perspective, the only way to address personal issues is to reduce work commitment, and the only way to have a fulfilling career is to make sacrifices in one's personal life. The compartmentalised view is an exclusive model, an 'either/or' model, whereby one must choose between the different priorities in life. This gives rise to winners and losers, and forces a choice between work and home life.

However, if an individual adopts the integrated view, work and personal life can support each other. They become part of the same integrated process that supports the overall mission in life. The concept is simple and the application need not be difficult. Employment provides income, which enables individuals to purchase goods and pursue activities that support other areas of their lives. Similarly, an individual who gains satisfaction and fulfilment at work will be a happier person at home at the end of the day. Conversely, those who are distracted from their work by an unhappy home life are unlikely to function effectively in the office. This approach can therefore produce a win–win situation in which the employee gains through a more fulfilling life and the employer benefits through increased energy, creativity and productivity brought to the job.

Perception is critical, and different individuals can see the same situation in opposite ways, with profound consequences for their lives. Expectation is a powerful force and expectations about ourselves tend to be self-fulfilling promises. Individuals who believe that success is not possible for them will not even see the opportunities which exist. Similarly, those who choose to adopt the compartmentalised view of life will condemn themselves to a state of conflict and stress.

Mahatma Gandhi said, 'One man cannot do right in one department of life whilst he is occupied doing wrong in any other department. Life is one indivisible whole.' These concepts are not new, but modern society seems to have forgotten that life is essentially a seamless entity rather than a series of discrete compartments. Building on Gandhi's teaching, employees cannot possibly perform consistently to their maximum potential if they are not addressing all aspects of their lives.

Effective pressure management

Pressure management is another key element in maintaining mental well-being. Most people need pressure, in the form of stimulation, motivation and challenge, to achieve their full potential. Pressure can have very positive effects, leading to success and personal growth, when individuals adapt successfully to the challenges they face. However, pressure which is excessive or which overloads coping mechanisms can have very negative effects, leading to stress, distress, impaired performance and ill health.

One widely used model of pressure management starts with pressure as the stimulus (Williams, 1994). This is the 'given' in the equation and is neither positive nor negative, but neutral. Successful adaptation to pressure leads to achievement, whereas failure to adapt gives rise to stress. The key to success relies upon learning and practising the attitudes and strategies that enable us consistently to produce a positive response. Responses, like all behaviours, can be learned and are not preordained. The skills of resilience increase the likelihood that pressure will lead to positive rather than negative consequences.

Another way of looking at this pressure management model is to imagine a balance mechanism, with resilience (or personality) as the fulcrum, modifying the response (see Figure 8.1, p. 62). The counterbalancing forces are sources of pressure on the one hand and the individual's coping mechanisms on the other. When individuals perceive the sources of pressure upon them as being greater than their ability to cope, they experience the negative effects of pressure. The resultant stress, with its attendant impairment of performance and loss of control, becomes a further source of pressure, giving rise to a self-reinforcing downward spiral – a vicious cycle. By contrast, when individuals perceive their coping mechanisms to be stronger than the sources of pressure upon them, the resulting growth and success lead to increased self-confidence, which in turn strengthens the coping mechanisms already in place, giving rise to a self-reinforcing upward spiral – a virtuous cycle.

The relationship between pressure, stress and resilience can be represented graphically (Figure 9.1). At the start of the curves, the relationship between pressure and performance is direct and linear. However, for any given individual, a point is reached where increasing pressure leads to a precipitate decrease in performance. This is the area of breakdown and burnout. The key to avoiding ill health is to maintain a position comfortably back from the edge of the precipice, so that there is a reserve to meet sudden unexpected demands. Runners can sprint only in short bursts, and there is a critical distinction between optimum pressure and maximum pressure. Nevertheless, the fact remains that organisations are looking to their employees for peak performance under high pressure. How can this be achieved without causing stress, breakdown and burnout?

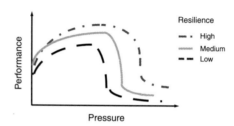

Figure 9.1 The relationship between pressure and performance, and its dependence on individual resilience.

The entire pressure–performance curve can be shifted upwards and to the right by increasing resilience. This enables individuals to perform better at any given level of pressure and to manage more pressure while staying away from the edge of the precipice. There is therefore benefit in providing tools and interventions which help people to move themselves from the lower to higher curves and, consequently, to higher and safer levels of performance for a given degree of pressure. Individuals who manage pressure effectively do not become stressed. Learning and practising effective behaviours, attitudes and strategies can help people to manage stress right out of their lives.

The organisational component

The role of the individual in maintaining balance and maximising personal growth is critical, but it is not the whole story. To return to the analogy of the tree: the tree grows in soil and the soil can be taken to represent the organisation. A tree will not grow to be healthy and strong in poor soil; likewise, organisational characteristics have an important bearing on the well-being of employees. Successful employers encourage high levels of personal capability, which in turn translate into high levels of organisational capability.

These desirable organisational features include:

- empowerment
- proactive change management
- respect/dignity
- supportive management and leadership styles
- balance-supportive culture
- flexibility/flexible working
- open, honest culture/trust
- active pursuit of win–win situations.

Resilient employees will use their skills to the greater benefit of the organisation for which they work only if the culture and the leadership style prevailing in that organisation are appropriate and conducive. Personal resilience, a supportive culture and empowering leadership are the three key prerequisites of outstanding organisational capability (Figure 9.2).

Conclusion

Most businesses now operate in a global market and success increasingly depends on individuals and teams achieving peak performance. Striking a sensible home/work balance is now widely recognised as being a critical success factor, and individuals who neglect this run the

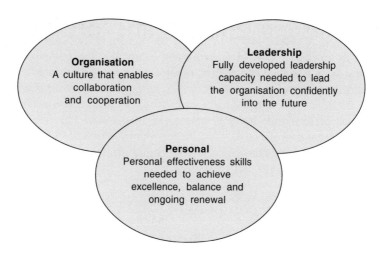

Figure 9.2 The three prerequisites of organisational capability.

long-term risk of impaired health. Organisations also need to foster a balanced view of work and personal life, in order to safeguard the interests not only of their employees but also of their shareholders.

References

Conner, D. R. (1995) *Managing at the Speed of Change*. New York: Villard Books.
Covey, S. R., Merrill, A. R. & Merrill, R. R. (1995) *First Things First*. New York: Simon and Schuster.
Seligman, M. (1992) *Learned Optimism*. New York: Random House.
Williams, S. (1994) *Managing Pressure for Peak Performance: The Positive Approach to Stress*. London: Kogan Page.

CHAPTER 10

Assessing mental health problems in the workplace

Matthew Hotopf and Janet Carruthers

Introduction

Assessing patients with psychiatric disorder requires time and skill. This chapter summarises some key elements of history taking and the mental state examination which we believe are important in occupational settings.

The most common psychiatric disorders in the general population and most medical settings are depression and anxiety. In occupational settings, substance misuse (including alcohol dependence) assumes special importance. Occupational physicians have to deal with the occasional employee who becomes acutely schizophrenic or manic. Patients with dementia or other organic psychiatric disorders are generally uncommon but may cause diagnostic problems. Diffuse disorders such as 'stress' are common presenting symptoms, and the task then is to determine whether a specific psychiatric disorder exits.

The clinical interview

The standard psychiatric assessment interview takes at least one hour and often longer. In occupational settings, more than one interview may be necessary to establish the nature and severity of the presenting disorder. The aims of the initial assessment are to establish rapport with the patient, to gain an understanding of the main complaints, examine potential causes and reach a preliminary diagnosis. In further interviews the occupational physician should aim to get a better understanding of causal factors, the patient's background and specific occupational factors which may have been influential.

The setting of the interview is important (Box 10.1): the physician should appear to be unhurried even though time is inevitably limited. As with most medical interviewing, the best approach is to start with relatively open questions and then move to clarify areas with narrower questions. Psychiatric history taking often involves gaining evidence

---

Box 10.1 Preliminaries for the clinical interview

- Use a private room.
- Appear unhurried.
- Interview with another staff member if there is any question of violence.
- Let the patient know how long you have available.
- Start by using open questions, for example 'What are the problems that brought you to see me?'
- Move on to closed questions to clarify specific topics, for example 'When did these feelings begin?', 'What do you think caused these problems?'
- Be clear with the patient about limits of confidentiality.
- Gain additional information from informants (family members, general practitioner, colleagues).
- Be prepared to arrange further interview if necessary.

---

from informants, especially for patients with poor insight. Colleagues can often give a good description of the character and duration of behavioural changes. The occupational physician may also wish to contact family members, and liaise with the general practitioner – with the employee's consent. The key headings for psychiatric history taking are shown in Box 10.2.

Confidentiality

It is important that the occupational physician reassures the employee of the confidential nature of the clinical discussion and that medical reports from the employee's general practitioner or consultant cannot be obtained without that employee's written consent. The occupational

---

Box 10.2 The psychiatric history

- Presenting complaints: onset, duration, pattern, triggering factors and consequences.
- Past psychiatric history: diagnosis and treatments.
- Past medical history.
- Family history: history of psychiatric disorder and descriptions of relationships in family.
- Personal history: childhood, education, relationships, forensic history.
- Occupational history: workplace exposures – organic and psychosocial.
- Alcohol and drugs.
- Current circumstances.
- Premorbid personality.

---

physician should also explain the employee's right to ask to see the report before it is sent to the occupational physician. Reports to management, by the occupational physician, should clarify the employee's ability to work and explain clearly any limitations of duties or working hours, and the proposal for clinical review during the rehabilitation period. If employees do not give consent to the physician to inform management about their medical condition, and the safety of the employee or colleagues is likely to be jeopardised by a return to work, the occupational physician has the right to breach confidentiality to protect the safety of others.

Specific occupational factors in the history

Occupational exposures should be carefully enquired after, especially for a first episode of psychosis or organic disorder. Traditionally recognised occupational risk factors have been organic ones such as tetra-ethyl lead. These are rare but vital to recognise as their removal may completely reverse serious disorders such as cognitive impairment and frank delirium or dementia. Some of the toxins workers may be exposed to and their consequences for mental health are listed in Table 10.1.

Stress in the workplace

Many employees will attribute an episode of depression or anxiety to work-related stress. Stress is a notoriously ambiguous term but it is gaining increasing importance, given recent lawsuits for the psychiatric consequences of stress. When assessing alleged work-related stress, it is worth asking a series of questions and documenting them carefully in the notes:

(1) Are there other pressures which the patient has failed to mention (e.g. a recent bereavement, marital breakdown or house move)?

Table 10.1 Occupational toxins and psychiatric disorders

Toxin	Mental health consequences of exposure
Solvents	Toxic confusional states and encephalopathies
Lead	Lead encephalopathy, dementia, psychosis
Tetra-ethyl lead	Acute psychosis, delirium, chronic fatigue and anxiety states
Mercury	'Erythism' – social avoidance and nervousness
Manganese	Headache, impotence, persistent laughter or tearfulness, impulsivity, acute psychosis
Thallium	Impaired consciousness, paranoia and depression
Carbon disulphide	Personality change, mood swings

Patients visiting occupational physicians may limit the discussion to workplace factors, while their general practitioner may have gained a very different understanding. Therefore it is important that occupational physicians and general practitioners communicate. Family and extra-work relationships are often powerful factors, while isolated work-related pressure is probably a relatively infrequent cause of psychiatric disorder. One or the other may be the final source of pressure which leads to the breakdown.

(2)   Is the pressure related to a specific problem (e.g. bullying by a manager) or does it refer to a non-specific complaint of overwork, frustration or boredom?

(3)   Does the source of work-related stress represent a genuine hardship or is it a symptom of psychiatric disorder? Employees who feel bullied by managers may have paranoid delusions. Those who feel overworked may be failing due to depression.

The mental state examination

The purpose of the mental state examination is to describe the appearance and behaviour of the individual and gain an understanding of current mood, experiences, thoughts and insight. The chief headings of the mental state examination are given in Box 10.3. The mental state is the key to reaching a diagnosis and assessing the severity of the disorder, and assessing the likelihood that the patient will comply with further management and treatment.

Assessing risk

Assessing risk behaviours is notoriously difficult; however, the psychiatric assessment should include a comment about the risk patients may represent to themselves or others. Assessing suicide risk involves a graded approach of asking questions from the least threatening to more specific and direct ones (Box 10.4). Assessing risk to others is less straightforward and involves a consideration of any previous history of violence or aggression, current mental state, insight and diagnosis.

Reaching a diagnosis

Psychiatric diagnosis uses a hierarchical system. At the top of the hierarchy are the organic disorders – for example, delirium and dementia and the neuropsychiatric consequences of substance misuse. Below these are psychotic disorders such as schizophrenia. Next come bipolar affective disorder (i.e. manic–depressive illness), and then depression and anxiety. Finally there is personality disorder. As the hierarchy is

---

Box 10.3 The mental state examination

Appearance and behaviour
- Hostile?
- Irritable?
- Threatening?
- Restless?
- Dishevelled?
- Smelling of alcohol?
- Suspicious?

Talk
- Rate and rhythm.
- Can the talk be readily understood?
- Is the speech slow or rapid?
- Does the talk have the usual modulation or is it flat and dull?

Mood
- Describe your general view of the patient's mood and the patient's own assessment. Do they agree?
- Experience of mood: feeling depressed and sad, or elated and high?
- Cognitive aspects of mood: self-esteem, view of future, helplessness, hopelessness, worthlessness, poor concentration.
- Biological aspects of mood: sleep, appetite, libido, energy.
- Suicidal ideas and plans.

Thoughts
- Form of thoughts: is speech understandable?
- Content of thoughts, including delusions or obsessions.

Perceptions
- Especially abnormal experiences such as hallucinations.

Cognitive assessment
- Orientation in time, place and person.
- Digit span.
- Short-term memory.
- Apraxias and agnosias.

Insight
- Does the patient understand he/she is unwell?
- Does the patient link phenomena (e.g. hallucinations and delusions) to illness?
- Is the patient prepared to be treated?

---

descended, the syndromes become less clear cut and more likely to merge with normality. Implicit in this system is the view that certain phenomena take precedence over others: more weight is given to disordered cognition than to hallucinations, or to depressed mood than to anxiety. If there is good evidence of delirium, this 'trumps' all other psychiatric diagnoses: therefore schizophrenia cannot be diagnosed

---

Box 10.4 Asking questions about suicide

- Start with broad, unthreatening remarks, such as 'Things seem to have been pretty bad recently. Do you sometimes feel hopeless?'
- Then move on to thoughts about dying passively: 'Do you sometimes not want to wake up in the morning?' or 'Is life worth living?'
- Then move on to questions more specifically about suicidal thoughts: 'Have you thought of harming yourself?'
- Finally, deal with specific details regarding plans: 'What have you considered doing? How far have you gone with this? What has stopped you?'

---

when delusions and hallucinations are thought to be due to delirium. Similarly, neurotic disorders cannot explain psychotic phenomena, but schizophrenia may be associated with neurotic symptoms (for example, anxiety).

Theoretically the diagnostic process should start at the top of the hierarchy (does the patient have delirium or dementia?) and work its way down through the hierarchy via psychosis, affective disorders and so on (Box 10.5).

When to refer

The decision on whom to refer to a psychiatrist will depend on the individual occupational physician's expertise and the degree to which

---

Box 10.5 Key questions in diagnosis

(1) Does the patient have an organic disorder?
- Signs of frank delirium or chronic global impairments associated with dementia.
- Psychotic phenomena may be present, but hallucinations are typically visual.

(2) Does the patient have a psychotic disorder?
- Hallucinations, delusions and thought disorder, with lack of insight.
- Phenomena may be denied but there will be evidence of bizarre behaviour.

(3) Does the patient have an affective disorder? Is the patient depressed or manic?
- Mania is elated mood and increased activity, whether mental or physical.
- Depression is indicated by low mood, biological symptoms and cognitive aspects such as hopelessness and guilt.

(4) Does the patient have a recognisable anxiety disorder: phobia, obsessive–compulsive disorder, generalised anxiety disorder or panic disorder?

> **Box 10.6** Types of problems appropriate for referral
>
> - Any organic disorders (at working age dementia should be referred to a neurologist).
> - Any psychotic disorders.
> - Mania.
> - Severe depression; depression associated with suicidal ideas; treatment-resistant depression.
> - Severe or treatment-resistant anxiety disorders.
> - Persistent suicidal ideas.
> - Patients with drug and alcohol problems if motivated to comply.

the employee represents a management problem. Box 10.6 indicates some of the types of problems which may be appropriate for referral but there are few hard-and-fast rules. Organic disorders, schizophrenia and mania presenting for the first time require adequate work-up by a specialist (which in the case of dementia in a patient of working age should be a neurologist). Uncomplicated cases of depression and neurotic disorders may not need specialist referral; however, patients whose conditions are resistant to treatment and those who have severe symptoms which raise concerns about self-harm should be referred. Referral for substance misuse is likely to depend more on the degree to which the patient is prepared to cooperate, and it may be necessary to reach a contract, one component of which would be compliance with specialist referral.

Many workplaces now have access to counsellors, whose training and expertise may vary. The occupational physician should be aware of the level of their expertise and if possible have agreed plans of action in case of serious disorders, such as psychotic illness, suicidal behaviour and behaviours which put others at risk. Such a plan of action should be made available to the entire occupational health team to ensure that inappropriate referral is avoided.

Further reading

Davies, T. (1997) Mental health assessment. *British Medical Journal*, **314**, 1536–1539.

Gelder, M., Gath, D. & Mayou, R. (1994) *Oxford Textbook of Psychiatry*. Oxford: Oxford University Press.

Institute of Psychiatry (1987) *Psychiatric Examination: Notes on Eliciting and Recording Clinical Information in Psychiatric Patients*. Oxford: Oxford University Press.

CHAPTER 11

Anxiety, depression, suicide risk, bullying and occupational health interventions

Maurice Lipsedge and Anne Margaret Samuel

Introduction

In the occupational health setting, just as in primary care, many people will seek medical help on the basis of physical symptoms when in reality there is an underlying psychiatric disorder. *Somatisation* is a useful concept. It covers situations where people seek help for somatic symptoms which they themselves erroneously attribute to an underlying physical disorder, when in fact a specific psychiatric illness, generally anxiety or depression (or both) is responsible. Employees may present to an occupational health department with a physical symptom rather than an emotional problem because of the widespread belief that physical symptoms are more acceptable to health care staff.

Anxiety

Anxiety is an experience familiar to everybody. People feel anxious before examinations and interviews, when their children return home late or when they have a near miss when driving. Anxiety is a normal short-term reaction to threat or danger and it prepares the individual for a physical response, namely fight or flight from the perceived threat.

The three questions to ask about a patient who may be suffering from an anxiety state are:

(1) Is the anxiety continuous or intermittent?
(2) Does the anxiety occur only in certain situations?
(3) Is the patient depressed as well as anxious?

Persistent anxiety

When the anxiety is more or less continuous, the diagnostic term 'generalised anxiety disorder' is used. This condition occurs in about 6% of the general population, and women are affected twice as often as men.

Patients will generally present with physical symptoms which indicate overactivity of the autonomic nervous system: palpitations, rapid heart beat, increased muscle tension (which can often cause headaches – 'a tight band around the head'), excessive sweating, pins and needles, faintness, dizziness, shakiness, epigastric discomfort and sometimes nausea or diarrhoea. They may also present with dysphagia, insomnia, fatigue or poor concentration. They will worry that one or more of their physical symptoms may have a sinister implication, and there may be fear of heart disease, cancer, AIDS and so on.

An employee may seek help for a single somatic symptom, such as difficulty in swallowing. Other somatic symptoms of anxiety, together with apprehensiveness and excessive worry, will confirm a diagnosis of anxiety. In addition to undue worry about health, a prominent psychological feature is endless concern about both major and trivial problems and excessive anxiety about coping with everyday situations and interactions with people, including colleagues, subordinates and supervisors, as well as with clients and other members of the public. Patients may also feel unreal or complain that their surroundings appear to be unfamiliar (termed 'depersonalisation' and 'derealisation', respectively).

Causative factors

When assessing a patient with anxiety (and/or depression) it is useful to classify causative factors into those that are:

(1) predisposing
(2) precipitating
(3) maintaining.

Predisposing factors include a vulnerable personality characterised by obsessionality or fear of rejection and of negative evaluation. There may be a genetic predisposition or childhood experience of rejection, separation or abuse. Another childhood influence may be the modelling effect of overanxious parents. It is useful to distinguish between *trait* anxiety, which is a lifelong anxious disposition, and *state* anxiety, which is a discrete episode.

Precipitating factors include major adverse life events. Anxiety is often triggered by threatened loss of status, job or security. (Depression tends to be a reaction to an established loss.) A potent cause of anxiety is severe short-term stress, especially when this involves a conflict of loyalties such as commitment to the employer versus responsibility for children, spouse or other relatives.

Maintaining (or perpetuating) factors include an intolerable situation at work, such as a combination of bullying and the imposition of unrealistic targets coupled with inadequate resources.

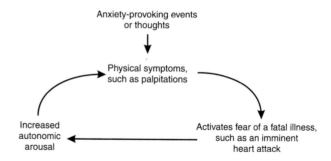

Figure 11.1 The cognitive model of acute anxiety (based on Salkovskis, 1992).

Panic disorder

This consists of discrete episodes of intense anxiety with an abrupt onset occurring several times a month. Each paroxysmal attack lasts for at least several minutes and, as with generalised anxiety disorder, there are both psychological and somatic symptoms. The physical symptoms are virtually the same as in generalised anxiety disorder but they occur in an intense and concentrated form. Patients interpret these physical symptoms in a catastrophic manner, believing that they are about to have a fatal heart attack, an epileptic fit, a faint or become acutely psychotic. A vicious spiral rapidly develops in which the more frightened the patient becomes, the more pronounced are the physical symptoms (see Figure 11.1). Thus, in panic disorder, physical symptoms lead to catastrophic thoughts of serious illness or social embarrassment which in turn exacerbate the physical symptoms.

Panic disorder occurs in up to 3.5% of the population. Panic attacks can supervene on a pre-existing generalised anxiety state or depressive disorder and can coexist with agoraphobia. In the early stages of panic disorder, the attacks are not necessarily associated with a specific situation. The differential diagnosis is outlined in Box 11.1.

Case 11.1 Panic disorder
A 40-year-old labourer, employed by his firm for 20 years, presented to the occupational health department with a 10-year history of panic attacks, which had begun when he was committed to doing a great deal of overtime. He had become very upset that he rarely saw his wife and children. During the attacks he would feel very anxious and experience a choking sensation in his throat, and would hyperventilate and sweat profusely. His symptoms persisted, even after he sensibly reduced his hours of work and had some debt counselling.

He had been treated with lorazepam, to which he became addicted. From time to time he had tried coming off the drug but experienced such devastating choking sensations that he resumed it. Eventually he became so anxious about having cancer or suffering a heart attack that he started drinking heavily as a form of self-medication.

> **Box 11.1** Differential diagnosis of generalised anxiety and panic disorder
>
> (1) Depression
> Anxiety may frequently accompany depressive illness. The two conditions share many symptoms (see Box 11.2) and where anxiety and depression coexist, patients may need a combination of treatments (e.g. antidepressants and cognitive–behavioural therapy).
>
> (2) Alcohol abuse
>
> (3) Drugs
> - Excessive caffeine consumption.
> - Illicit drugs, especially amphetamine.
> - Withdrawal from a benzodiazepine (typically taken as a hypnotic or tranquilliser).
>
> (4) Physical conditions
> - Thyrotoxicosis.
> - Paroxysmal tachycardia.
> - Hypoglycaemia.
> - Temporal lobe epilepsy (ask about déjà vu and olfactory and gustatory hallucinations as well as marked depersonalisation and derealisation, and remember that epileptic phenomena are short-lived and intermittent rather than continuous).
> - Phaeochromocytoma is an extremely rare cause of symptoms that resemble panic attacks.

By the time he was seen he had a very high level of free-floating anxiety and a constant sense of apprehension, difficulty in relaxing and epigastric discomfort. He had had to give up his hobby of fishing due to intrusive ruminations about death while waiting for the fish to bite.

He was switched from lorazepam to diazepam (which has a longer half-life and makes eventual withdrawal easier) and was encouraged gradually to increase his physical exercise. He also had sessions of anxiety management with a clinical psychologist, and he learned to recognise the link between some of his worrying thoughts and his physical symptoms.

He responded well to this regime and was able to continue working.

Phobic anxiety disorders

Unlike other anxiety disorders, phobic anxiety occurs in specific situations (Table 11.1). There is an irrational fear and avoidance of specific objects or situations. Although sufferers recognise that their fear is excessive and inappropriate, they cannot be argued out of it. While *specific phobias*, such as a fear of certain small animals, are very common and rarely cause occupational disability, *agoraphobia*, which can merge with *travel phobia*, can cause significant occupational impairment. In agoraphobia the patient feels anxious in crowded places or open spaces, or places or situations from which escape would be difficult or

Table 11.1 Comparison of anxiety disorders in terms of duration and specificity to certain situations

	Duration	Situation specific?
Generalised anxiety disorder	Long	No
Panic attacks	Brief	No
Phobic anxiety	Brief	Yes

embarrassing, for example supermarket queues, traffic jams and public transport. Patients tend to feel safer in their own homes but in the most severe cases they insist that somebody is with them at all times.

Whereas agoraphobia tends to occur in young women, *social phobias* occur equally commonly in men and women. They include an intense fear of being scrutinised or evaluated by others. This may lead to avoidance of speaking or eating in public, conversing with strangers or of writing in the presence of others. Note that social phobia as well as generalised anxiety disorder, panic disorder and agoraphobia can all be associated with alcohol misuse.

Treatment of anxiety disorders

Physical examination

Physical examination may reveal an underlying physical cause, especially thyrotoxicosis, and also serves to reassure the patient.

Psychological treatment

- Explain the fight–flight mechanism – autonomic activity once had survival value but is counterproductive in contemporary life.
- Describe the inverted U-shape relationship between anxiety and performance.
- Explain the self-perpetuating vicious circle which links excessive worry to increased activity of the sympathetic nervous system.
- Help patients to devise a problem-solving approach to their difficulties.
- Provide tape-recorded instructions on relaxation techniques and arrange for anxiety management training.

The more intractable cases benefit from cognitive–behavioural therapy. The cognitive–behavioural therapy of agoraphobia includes graded exposure to the feared situation (see case 11.2), while training in social skills and assertiveness as well as cognitive–behavioural therapy are effective in the treatment of social phobias.

Case 11.2 Phobic anxiety

A 40-year-old delivery man presented to the occupational health department with symptoms of anxiety and frequency of micturition over the previous few months. He attributed the anxiety to the recent introduction of a new monitoring device which he found difficult to cope with because he thought his manager would be checking up on him. This made his bladder problem worse and he resorted to carrying a bottle with him during the day to save time finding a lavatory.

This man was suffering from 'sphincter phobia' – a fear of needing to go to the lavatory at inconvenient or embarrassing times. He responded well to behavioural psychotherapy. This involved being given two cups of tea at the start of each session and then being sent out to walk increasing distances, with a full bladder and without his bottle. He made good progress and was able to carry out his job without stopping to micturate more than once a morning, although he continued to carry his bottle with him for reassurance.

Pharmacological treatment

- Reserve benzodiazepines for the very short-term management of intense anxiety.
- Benzodiazepines can be invaluable in emergencies, when there is no risk of dependence.
- Benzodiazepines taken for more than two weeks can cause rebound anxiety and insomnia when the drug is withdrawn.
- Antidepressants, especially tricyclics, can help to relieve the symptoms of generalised anxiety – some patients become more anxious when taking a selective serotonin reuptake inhibitor (SSRI).
- Dothiepin has an anti-anxiety effect equivalent to that of a minor tranquilliser but is markedly cardiotoxic in overdose.
- Beta-blockers are helpful for the relief of pronounced tremor, which may contribute to social phobia.

Obsessional–compulsive disorder (OCD)

This disorder comprises ruminations (obsessions) and compulsive rituals. The ruminations consist of recurrent intrusive thoughts concerned with contamination, disease, blasphemy or distressing sexual or sadistic preoccupations. The commonest rituals consist of checking, cleaning and counting. The obsessions are unwelcome and many patients try to resist carrying out the rituals but are overwhelmed by the anxiety that resistance provokes. OCD is often associated with major depression and both clomipramine and SSRIs can be helpful, even in the absence of concurrent depression. The specific effect of clomipramine, which is a potent serotonin reuptake inhibitor, and of the SSRIs, suggests that serotonin has a role in the pathophysiology of OCD.

Obsessional ruminations are difficult to deal with by psychological means but compulsive rituals can be treated with a combination of exposure and response prevention.

The impact of OCD on productivity is self-evident. Endless checking and repetitions can lead to habitual lateness or lingering in the workplace at the end of the day. Patients with OCD are often ashamed and embarrassed about their symptoms, which may come to light only after a disciplinary procedure because of apparent inefficiency or incompetence. Thus, a postman caused numerous complaints from householders when he repeatedly returned to check that he had delivered the mail to the correct address.

Case 11.3 OCD

A 31-year-old apprentice presented with symptoms of anxiety and OCD. He had an obsessional previous personality, being a perfectionist, tidy and punctual. He had become almost paralysed by *folie de doute* when he spent an inordinate amount of time checking and rechecking terminals, switches, locks and so on, and he kept returning to his previous customer to confirm that he had carried out the job safely.

He underwent behavioural psychotherapy (a response-prevention programme) and was rehabilitated back to full-time work within six months.

Depressive disorders

Symptoms

The symptoms of depression can be divided into psychological and somatic. Psychological symptoms include persistent lowering of mood, with low self-esteem, pessimism, a sense of despair, hopelessness and helplessness, thoughts of suicide and irrational ideas of guilt and self-reproach. The somatic (biological) symptoms include loss of drive and energy. There is impairment of concentration, appetite, sleep and sex drive. Some patients eat excessively ('comfort eating').

There is also loss of a sense of enjoyment ('anhedonia'). The patient's mood may be significantly worse in the morning and improve somewhat as the day goes on (diurnal variation). The depression is classified as being of psychotic intensity when the patient experiences auditory hallucinations (typically making critical accusations) or has delusions of guilt. A formal diagnosis of depression requires the presence of the majority of the non-psychotic symptoms. However, patients may present with a somatic symptom such as backache and they themselves may not recognise that in fact they are suffering from a depressive illness.

Box 11.2 lists the symptoms that may appear in both depression and anxiety states.

Prevalance

The point prevalence of depressive illness is about 3% of men and up to 9% of women, with a lifetime risk in the general population of up to 12%

> **Box 11.2** Symptoms common to both anxiety and depression
>
> Impaired concentration
> Insomnia
> Loss of weight
> Loss of libido
> Non-specific physical symptoms, for example muscle tension
> Irritability
> Undue preoccupation with health
> Fatigue

for men and 26% for women. Nearly 1% of the population is at risk of bipolar affective disorder (manic–depressive disorder). Genetic factors predispose to mood disorders, as shown by the high rates of the more severe types of disorder in first-degree relatives of people with depression.

Risk factors

Social factors are of great importance as precipitants of depressive illness. Major adverse life events increase the risk of depression sixfold in the six months after the event. Other risk factors for depressive episodes, especially those following life events, include the loss of a parent before the age of 11 years and the lack of a confiding relationship with a partner.

Depression and alcohol misuse

Some patients with a primary depressive illness medicate themselves with alcohol. Conversely, alcoholics may go through bouts of depression that are precipitated by adverse changes in their social circumstances, while depression (and anxiety) can also occur during alcohol withdrawal (see Chapter 12 for a detailed description of the symptoms of alcohol dependence and withdrawal).

Depression and bereavement

Factors that increase the risk of developing a morbid or protracted grief reaction include death of a child or of a spouse, death that is sudden, unexpected, untimely or violent, and death for which the survivor feels responsible. Individuals are more at risk of pathological or protracted grief if they had an ambivalent or unduly dependent relationship with the deceased, if they have a history of mental health problems, if their family is perceived as unhelpful, or if there are other concurrent major adverse life events. When the relationship with the deceased has been ambivalent or full of conflict, feelings of guilt and anger complicate the course of grieving.

Those patients who develop a frank depressive illness may need an antidepressant. Antidepressants are also useful for patients who develop panic disorder as one of the psychiatric sequelae of bereavement. The voluntary organisation CRUSE is an invaluable counselling resource for the bereaved. Murray Parkes and Markus (1998), in a chapter on bereavement in adult life, provide helpful guidelines on understanding and helping people who have been bereaved.

The assessment of depression

The assessment of depression always requires an assessment of suicide risk (see below).

When investigating a first episode of depression it is important to look for a link between depression and physical illness or its treatment:

- corticosteroids and antihypertensive drugs, especially reserpine, methyldopa and levodopa, can cause depression
- depression can be a reaction to painful or potentially life-threatening physical disorders
- the symptoms of some physical illnesses, especially myxoedema (apathy, general slowing down, sluggishness, poor memory), resemble depression, and at yimes thyrotoxicosis, hyperparathyroidism and systemic lupus erythematosis can also present as depression
- depression may be a complication of other illnesses, for instance Parkinson's disease and Cushing's syndrome; it may also follow a viral infection, such as infectious mononucleosis and hepatitis.

Dysthymia

Dysthymia is a chronic depression of mood which does not fulfil the criteria of recurrent depressive disorder. Most of the time sufferers feel tired and miserable, although there are periods of days or weeks when they feel well and in general they can cope with the basic demands of everyday life. Dysthymia is commoner in women than in men and in the first-degree biological relatives of patients with a history of depressive episodes. Patients may benefit from antidepressants or cognitive therapy (see below).

Diagnostic tools

Beck Depression Inventory

This is a widely used self-rating inventory of proven validity, reliability and sensitivity to change. It comprises 21 items, each describing a specific behavioural manifestation of depression. Completion of the inventory results in a total score (maximum 63), which is a measure of the depth of depression (Beck *et al*, 1988a).

Beck Anxiety Inventory

This is a 21-item self-report inventory for measuring the severity of anxiety. It is recognised as a reliable and valid measure of anxiety which has high internal consistency and test–retest reliability as well as good concurrent and discriminant validity (Beck *et al*, 1988*b*).

Hospital Anxiety and Depression Scale

This scale, devised by Zigmond & Snaith (1983), comprises 14 items. It was designed specifically for use in non-psychiatric hospital departments. The items on the scale are all concerned with the psychological symptoms of neurosis, thus making it suitable for use in patients with concurrent physical illness and disabilities.

Treatment of depression

Psychological treatment

Patients with depression have a negative attitude to themselves, to the world around them and to their future. Cognitive therapy consists of the identification of negative autonomic thoughts and training the patient to challenge these distortions. Examples of distorted thinking include:

- selective abstraction ('I have not achieved my targets, so I am a useless employee')
- arbitrary inference ('my job must be at risk because my boss appeared angry with me today').

In mild to moderate depression, cognitive therapy is as effective as an antidepressant and it can also help to prevent further episodes of depression. A course of cognitive therapy consists of 12–20 sessions, each of one hour. The therapist elicits habitual distortions in thinking, teaches the patient to challenge these maladaptive thoughts and thus alter the processing of information which has been perpetuating the depressed mood. Cognitive therapy helps patients to modify the negative expectations, assumptions, rules and schemata that determine their view of themselves and their relationships.

Case 11.4 Major depression

A 40-year-old computer engineer presented with symptoms of depression. He had resigned from several jobs in the past while feeling like this and these episodes, which lasted from three to six months, recurred at three-yearly intervals. During these episodes he became preoccupied both professionally and personally with feelings of inadequacy. Despite a first-class university degree, he felt he was too slow to take in existing programmes and felt ill equipped on the technical side.

He described all the features of the 'impostor complex': he believed he had been overpromoted and was concerned that he would be exposed as a fraud; as a result he considered resigning.

He was treated with lofepramine and underwent cognitive therapy with a clinical psychologist to teach him ways of restoring his self-confidence as well as reassessing his skills to reinforce his capabilities. He made steady progress and, despite one minor relapse when he stopped the antidepressant prematurely, he is now off medication and is a much-valued employee.

Pharmacological treatment

In severe depression, antidepressants which potentiate both serotonin and noradrenaline transmission are the most effective (e.g. venlafaxine). In less severe depression, the tricyclics and SSRIs appear to be equally effective. All types of antidepressant have a latent interval of two weeks before the onset of a significant antidepressant effect, although the anti-anxiety effect (e.g. with a sedative tricyclic antidepressant such as dothiepin) is observed much earlier. Patients should be warned about the possibility of side-effects (e.g. dry mouth, constipation, drowsiness and postural hypotension with tricyclic antidepressants). They should also be told that the drugs are not addictive and that they must not expect an immediate response since recovery may take a matter of weeks. This should increase compliance.

Reasons for apparent treatment failure with antidepressants include starting at too high a dose, which causes intolerable side-effects and loss of compliance. Conversely, there is also a tendency to prescribe inadequate doses. The full therapeutic dose of tricyclics is at least 125 mg daily. The SSRIs may be better tolerated than tricyclic antidepressants and are safer when driving or using moving machinery.

In apparently treatment-resistant depression, the dose of antidepressants should be pushed up to the limits of tolerance and lithium can be used as an augmentor. The most severe cases of depression, including those of psychotic intensity, require electroconvulsive therapy (ECT).

The antidepressant should be continued for six months after recovery because about half the patients will relapse if the drug is stopped prematurely. Up to three-quarters of patients who have had an episode of major depression will suffer a relapse within ten years and perhaps 20% of patients with very severe depression become chronically depressed. The long-term administration of antidepressants can be helpful in preventing recurrent relapses.

Adverse effects of antidepressants

The adverse effects are brought about by blockade of post-synaptic neurotransmitter receptors. Tricyclic antidepressants block muscarinic, histamine and alpha$_1$-adrenoreceptors and can therefore cause:

* drowsiness and slowing of cognition
* dry mouth
* constipation
* weight gain

- tachycardia
- postural hypotension (and in overdose they can cause cardiac arrhythmias)
- dysuria
- erectile dysfunction
- blurred vision

Lofepramine is a modified tricyclic antidepressant which mainly affects noradrenaline uptake and it is relatively well tolerated.

The SSRIs block only serotonin reuptake. Common side-effects include:

- nausea
- anxiety
- insomnia
- erectile difficulties
- delayed orgasm.

Although venlafaxine blocks both noradrenaline and serotonin re-uptake, its adverse effect profile is like that of the SSRIs.

Diagnostic classification systems

There are two diagnostic classification systems: ICD–10 (World Health Organization, 1992) and DSM–IV (American Psychiatric Association, 1994). DSM–IV is more highly structured than ICD–10 and it gives clear operational rules on making diagnoses, whereas ICD–10 is more descriptive. The DSM–IV multi-axial system permits the separate evaluation of clinical disorders, personality disorders, mental retard-ation, general medical conditions, psychosocial and environmental problems and global assessment of functioning: that is, it emphasises the biopsychosocial model. Another advantage of DSM–IV over ICD–10 is that the diagnostic criteria include the social and occupational consequences of the disorder.

The two major ICD–10 groups which cover the topics of this chapter are mood (affective) disorders (F3) and the neurotic disorders (F4). (DSM–IV has replaced the word 'neurotic' with 'anxiety'.)

Deliberate self-harm and suicide

Deliberate self-poisoning is the commonest reason for the acute medical admission of women and the second commonest reason for the admission of men, after ischaemic heart disease. About 30 years ago self-harm occurred twice as commonly in women as in men but the female:male ratio has been significantly reduced. The commonest age group involved is under 35 years, especially adolescents and young adults. High-risk groups include the economically deprived residents of the inner cities. Single and divorced people are more at risk. Deliberate self-harm is statistically associated with the premature death of a parent and other types of childhood separation. Three-quarters of episodes of self-harm are precipitated by problematic relationships with partners. Those who carry out deliberate self-harm often lack parenting skills and self-harm occurs at least ten times more often among unemployed people than in those who have jobs. Other risk factors include general medical problems and epilepsy. The commonest psychiatric disorders found in patients who harm themselves are transient 'adjustment disorders', followed by depressive illness. Personality disorders and misuse of alcohol are also common.

The vast majority of self-harm is by poisoning, commonly with paracetamol, aspirin or hypnotics. Of other forms of self-harm, wrist-cutting is the commonest.

Many acts of deliberate self-harm are impulsive and patients will often say that they merely wished to go to sleep or to gain respite from distressing thoughts. There is often a mixture of *expressive* and *instrumental* motives: that is, patients wish to communicate their distress and also to influence people, such as partners, children or parents and sometimes employers.

Situations which trigger deliberate self-harm include relationship problems and difficulties with employment or studies, and financial worries.

About 15% of patients are involved in a further episode of deliberate self-harm within one year and 1% of patients actually kill themselves during that period.

Factors suggesting serious suicidal intent include:

- planning and preparations (hoarding of tablets and putting financial affairs in order)
- taking precautions to avoid discovery
- leaving a suicide note
- admitting that the aim of the self-harm was to cause death.

The ultimate risk of suicide in those who have harmed themselves is significantly increased in patients who evince a sense of marked hopelessness.

Older women, men, unemployment, people living alone, poor physical health, psychiatric disorder and a history of self-harm, especially if violent methods were used, are all pointers to an increased risk of suicide. A high degree of suicidal intent can be inferred from the use of a dangerous method such as hanging, electrocution, jumping or drowning. Most people who kill themselves have told someone of their intention and repeated attempts often eventually succeed. Multiple methods in the same attempt or violent methods suggest a strong wish to die.

Assessment of risk after deliberate self-harm

- Was the attempt concealed or openly revealed?
- Was it planned or impulsive?
- Was there a note?
- What was the patient's state of mind at the time of the attempt and leading up to it?
- Does the patient regret the failure of the attempt?
- Is the patient glad to be alive?
- Does the patient intend to try again?
- Is there a history of attempts?
- Is there a family history of suicide?
- Are there delusions of guilt or self-recrimination?
- Are there command hallucinations?
- Is there alcohol or drug misuse?
- Does the patient have any physical illness?
- Does the patient have social supports?
- Is the patient single, widowed, divorced or separated?
- Are there hypochondriacal delusions or delusions of unworthiness?

Caution

The decision to end one's life or the attempt to do so can have a cathartic effect, so the patient may appear surprisingly cheerful before or after an act of deliberate self-harm and this may give the impression that the depression has lifted or that there is no further risk.

Case 11.5 Suicide
A 50-year-old painter and decorator presented with a painful neck and shoulder following an injury sustained when he was struck by heavy scaffolding while working. Despite orthopaedic and neurological specialist advice and follow-up, he was left with intractable pain and was prevented from resuming his job or any other suitable alternative duties. He could also no longer engage in his hobby of weight-lifting, at which he had reached an international standard. He was given an antidepressant, but in a low dose.

After a year off work he made a serious suicide attempt. The dose of antidepressant was increased and further efforts were made to retrain him as the antidepressants became effective. He was also treated by a clinical psychologist specialising in chronic pain to teach him to cope with daily tasks despite a significant background level of pain. However, there was very little improvement and as he was unable to work he was retired on ill-health grounds. He committed suicide three months later.

Treatment of deliberate self-harm

After an act of deliberate self-harm:

- ensure the person's physical well-being with appropriate medical treatment

- evaluate the risk of the act being repeated
- arrange admission to a psychiatric unit for people with serious mental illness or people who still have suicidal intent
- arrange for brief problem-solving counselling sessions relevant to the individual's current life situation (Lipsedge, 1997).

Bullying

Bullying can cause both anxiety and depression. The following categories of bullying behaviour occur in the workplace:

- *threat to professional status*, such as belittling opinion
- *threat to personal standing*, such as devaluing with reference to age
- *isolation*, for example by the withholding of information
- *overwork*, for example by the imposition of impossible deadlines
- *destabilisation*, for example by removal of responsibility on the one hand or setting up to fail on the other (Rayner, 1997).

Bullied employees tend to be diagnosed as suffering from 'stress' or as being involved in a 'clash of personalities', so the blame is located within the victim rather than in the psychosocial work environment. The most damaging form of bullying – the one that is most likely to cause psychological ill health and so lead to absenteeism – is criticising the individual's private life or repeatedly mocking a handicap or mannerism. The overall impact of bullying is that victims feel harassed and their work is adversely affected. Research in Sweden has shown that a significant proportion of people who commit suicide have a history of being bullied at work (Leymann, 1996). Some victims of bullying, exposed to repeated negative experiences, may fall into the state of apathy and resignation known as 'learned helplessness'.

Some organisations have an anti-bullying policy based on the recognition that bullying can have widespread disruptive effects within the workplace.

Occupational health interventions

As an example of an organisational initiative taken to address mental ill-health issues, London Electricity has implemented an occupational health risk management programme. The approach is described in detail in Chapter 3. In summary, it includes:

(1) *A management of mental health module* geared towards helping managers and supervisors to identify behavioural changes in their employees and if a mental health problem is suspected, to provide sufficient support while directing the employee towards the occupational health department.

(2) *An ergonomics risk management module* aimed at avoiding a mismatch between the employees' skills and tasks and identifying potential hazards such as job and workstation design, so that any resulting risks can be assessed and controlled.

(3) *Developing close links with psychological and psychiatric specialists* through:

- conducting a stress audit
- introducing a rapid response
- a trauma counselling programme
- formal psychiatric assessment of all employees with long-term sickness absence with a diagnosis of depression, anxiety, 'ME' (myalgic encephalomyelitis), chronic fatigue, post-viral state, 'stress', 'burnout', and so on.

(4) *Training in change management techniques.*

(5) Developing a confidential self-referral system, that is, an *employee support programme.*

In this particular organisation sickness absence due to mental ill health is falling, and the number of mental ill health retirement cases fell between the years 1994/95 and 1996/97. The early detection and energetic treatment of depression and anxiety disorders can greatly reduce both sickness absence and the likelihood of ill health retirement.

References

American Psychiatric Association (1994) *Diagnostic and Statistical Manual of Mental Disorders* (4th edn) (DSM–IV). Washington, DC: APA.

Beck, A. T., Steer, R. A. & Garbin, M. G. (1988a) Psychometric properties of the Beck Depression Inventory: 25 years later. *Clinical Psychology Review*, **8**, 77–100.

—, Epstein, N., Brown, G., *et al* (1988b) An inventory for measuring clinical anxiety: psychometric properties. *Journal of Consulting and Clinical Psychology*, **6**, 893–897.

Leymann, H. (1996) Sjalvmord till foljd av forhallanden i arbetsmiljon [Suicide and conditions in the workplace]. *Arbete Manniska Miljo*, **3**, 155–160.

Lipsedge, M. (1997) Suicide and deliberate self-harm. In *Textbook of Psychiatry* (eds L. Rees, M. Lipsedge & C. Ball). London: Arnold.

Murray Parkes, C. & Markus, A. (1998) *Coping with Loss: Helping Patients and Their Families*. London: BMJ Books.

Rayner, C. (1997) The incidence of workplace bullying. *Journal of Community and Applied Social Psychology*, **3**, 199–208.

Salkovskis, P. (1992) The cognitive–behavioural approach. In *Medical Symptoms not Explained by Organic Disease* (eds F. Creed, R. Mayou & A. Hopkins), pp. 70–84. London: Royal College of Psychiatrists and Royal College of Physicians of London.

World Health Organization (1992) *Tenth Revision of the International Classification of Diseases* (ICD–10). Geneva: WHO.

Zigmond, A. S. & Snaith, R. P. (1983) The Hospital Anxiety and Depression Scale. *Acta Psychiatrica Scandinavica*, **67**, 361–370.

CHAPTER 12

Substance misuse/addiction: alcohol

Paul Gwinner and David Moore

Introduction

Alcohol is a drug. Only about 10% of the British population are teetotal. Two-thirds of men and one-third of women drink regularly. Most people who drink alcohol, however, do so without harm and only a minority of drinkers develop a problem. Of those who do, most remain in employment and their drinking will impinge on the workplace. Occupational physicians and managers therefore need to know the risks or factors that may make a drinker more vulnerable to developing a problem.

Impact on work

Although there are famous instances of gifted individuals performing spectacularly well despite heavy drinking, alcohol misuse has a substantial collective adverse effect upon a person's ability to work. The effects may be summarised as impaired working relationships, accidents, waste of productive time and resources, and suboptimal productivity. A person's alcohol misuse also may affect colleagues, and thereby reduce morale, and, indeed, collusion may occur, where colleagues cover for the person affected. These factors combine, imposing a cost on the employing organisation and community alike. There is no entirely satisfactory basis for the computation of the overall cost to industry: the best available estimate, of £1.7 billion, dates from 1987 and includes direct and indirect costs. Difficulties in the estimation of such global figures do not preclude individual cost–benefit analysis in the evaluation of workplace action to minimise the problem in any one organisation.

The direct effects of alcohol at work include:

- accidents
- poor quality work
- dishonesty
- poor-quality decision-making

- lateness
- harassment
- absenteeism
- 'presenteeism'
- sickness absence
- disruptive behaviour
- employee relations difficulties
- incurred legal liability
- driving offences.

Individual factors

As Table 12.1 indicates, factors in the development of drinking problems are usually multiple.

Occupational risk factors

People who misuse alcohol may be attracted into an occupational grouping where many of the factors listed below operate:

- availability and accessibility of alcohol in the workplace
- traditions of drinking at work
- corporate entertainment
- freedom from supervision
- separation from family
- all-male work.

Table 12.1 Individual risk factors for developing drinking problems

Factor	Effect
Gender	Men are twice as likely to develop a drinking problem as women. An increasing number of women, however, are developing drinking problems.
Culture	Certain cultural groups have a higher incidence of drinking problems.
Personality	Those with high levels of anxiety and individuals prone to depression are particularly susceptible to drinking problems.
Social factors	People who are socially isolated or divorced and those who have been recently bereaved are recognised as vulnerable to the development of alcohol problems. Those from a domestic or family background of heavy drinking are also at risk.
Habit	Those who establish a habit of frequent heavy alcohol consumption are at greater risk of developing a serious drinking problem.

Individual occupational risks

The following categories are particularly at risk of problem drinking:

- the highly stressed senior executive
- the potentially redundant ageing manager
- the anxious but over-promoted employee
- the professionally bored employee
- the unsupervised worker
- the professionally isolated employee
- the middle-aged employee resistant to organisational/cultural change
- those frequently absent from home on business
- the expatriate employee
- those workers whose jobs involve heavy manual labour, particularly in grossly uncomfortable working environments.

Indicators of problematic drinking in the workplace

- Frequently smelling of alcohol at work.
- Drunkenness at work.
- Accidents suffered by the employee associated with drinking.
- Deteriorating professional proficiency.
- Poor sickness absence record.
- Often short spells of self-certified sickness after weekends or public holidays.
- Reputation in the workforce as a 'steady heavy'.
- Evidence of withdrawal symptoms.
- Drinking and driving charges – particularly in those employees whose employment depends on maintaining a clean licence.
- Inappropriately heavy consumption of alcohol at company events.
- Domestic problems.
- Instability of mood in the course of the working day often associated with irritability and emotional disinhibition.

Characteristics of alcohol problems

Alcohol problems are protean. In the workplace the individual employee with a drink problem can therefore present in a number of ways. These can be represented broadly by a simple model (Figure 12.1).

Treatment and intervention

- Occupational health staff should not be responsible for the primary treatment of the person who is misusing alcohol.

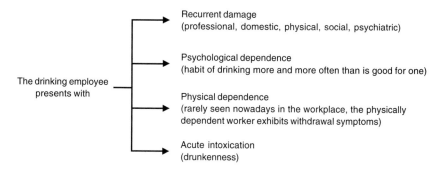

Figure 12.1 A simple model of the presentation of alcohol problems in an employee.

- The role of the occupational physician is essentially one of monitoring, providing fitness-to-work assessments and providing advice to management about job modification and support for the person with a drinking problem.
- There is a range of treatment options (e.g. individual counselling, group work, residential rehabilitation, day programmes and detoxification) but no single treatment model is successful with all people who misuse alcohol. The physically dependent drinker will invariably require detoxification. This is usually done as an in-patient, although it is now increasingly undertaken in the community. Employees being detoxified should not be allowed to be at work.
- Approximately one-third of people who misuse alcohol recover without treatment.

Treatment goals

Total abstinence is the treatment goal of choice for the person who has sustained serious physical damaged through the misuse of alcohol, who is physically dependent on alcohol or who has tried to maintain controlled drinking but has failed.

Controlled drinking may be an acceptable treatment goal for someone who is non-dependent and physically undamaged and who has not yet established major problems as a consequence of drinking. Controlled drinking is more likely to be an attainable goal if an abstinent state of several months has first been established.

Some people with a drinking problem can be helped by deterrent drug therapy using disulfiram (Antabuse).

Brief intervention

Brief intervention (usually provided by general practitioners) should include simple education about drinking, assessment of alcohol intake, advice on how to reduce intake and motivational interviewing. This intervention has been shown to be as effective as specialist intervention.

Local services

Occupational health staff should be aware of local services geographically accessible to the workplace and how to contact them. They may include:

- a community alcohol team (CAT)
- in-patient facilities (both private and in the public sector)
- local councils on alcohol
- alcohol information or advisory services (listed in the telephone directory)
- the self-help groups Alcoholics Anonymous and Al-Anon.

Do not forget

- The general practitioner and the community psychiatric nurse can provide effective services.
- Early intervention is often more successful in terms of treatment outcome than late intervention.
- Occupational health staff should always encourage management to intervene early with an employee with a drinking problem.
- Many early signs of problem drinking are behavioural rather than medical, and will therefore impinge on management first.
- Occupational health departments should include alcohol and drinking problems as part of health promotion activities.
- Educational material about alcohol and drinking problems should be available and accessible to the workforce in occupational health departments.
- Occupational health staff should always enquire about drinking when assessing or seeing patients.

Prevention in the workplace

Preventive action can include:

- a statement on drinking at work
- an alcohol policy (to include safe levels, legal duties, random testing)
- management education
- health education on the effects of alcohol on performance, accidents and health.

Prevention starts with a policy statement on alcohol consumption at work applicable to all employees and with explicit penalties for

---

Box 12.1 Policy on alcohol

The policy must:
- be confidential
- apply to *all* employees.

The employer undertakes:
- to suspend any disciplinary action related to alcohol misuse
- to guarantee the employee's job or equivalent
- to provide time off for treatment with normal benefits
- to guarantee confidentiality.

The drinking employee undertakes:
- to acknowledge the problem
- to accept, comply with and respond to advice or treatment.

---

non-compliance (see Box 12.1). This does not necessarily mean a 'dry site'. This statement may be the preamble to, or setting for, a formal policy on alcohol, encouraging drinking employees to seek help.

Managers need training in the recognition and management of employees who are misusing alcohol. This should include the operation of the company alcohol policy. All employees, irrespective of grade, should be given training on the effects of alcohol misuse with regard to performance, accident risk and health, and the existence and provisions of the company alcohol policy. 'Safe levels' of consumption should be emphasised, remembering that in some circumstances drinking at a 'safe level' may still be inappropriate. Employees must be reminded of their duties under legislation, especially the Road Traffic and the Health and Safety at Work etc. Act. In some industries and occupations, for example public transport, alcohol misuse may legally be determined by random breath testing. These actions should form part of a coherent programme with both management and employee support. It must be a continuing programme and considerable ingenuity may be needed to keep it 'fresh'.

Management in the workplace

Formal policies on alcohol are a reasonably effective way of managing the problem of alcohol misuse in an employing organisation by helping employees with a drinking problem and minimising the potential for employee relations difficulties. In essence, they represent an explicit contract between the employer and employees of all grades that the organisation will not penalise alcohol-related poor work or indiscipline, provided that the drinker admits misuse, accepts help and benefits from it. The 'contract' is confidential and will include the employer's promise to arrange or provide help, to allow 'time off' for treatment under normal sick pay arrangements and, most importantly, a job guarantee. The formal policy must be supported by detailed procedures covering definitions, criteria, responsibilities and administration.

Some organisations use an employee assistance programme. The programme effectively guarantees confidentiality by removing the management of the problem to an outside agency. Again, such a programme requires detailed supporting procedures within the organisation. They are expensive, although cost–benefit is claimed.

Further reading

Alcohol Services Directory 1998/9 (available through Alcohol Concern: tel. 020 7928 7377)

Cooper, C. & Williams, S. (eds) (1994) *Creating Healthy Work Organisations*. Chichester: John Wiley & Sons.

Hutcheson, G. D., Henderson, M. M. & Davies, J. B. (1995) *Alcohol in the Workplace: Costs and Responses*. London: Department for Education and Employment.

CHAPTER 13

Substance misuse/addiction: drugs

C. C. H. Cook and Graham Bell

Causative factors

Misuse of drugs is an increasing public issue. About 28% of 12- to 59-year-olds have used an illicit drug at some time in their lives (Institute for the Study of Drug Dependence, 1997) and about one-third of these people have done so in the past year. However, there is an upward trend in such statistics, and as drugs are more widely used and misused, we must expect to encounter them with increasing regularity in the workplace.

The aetiology is multifactorial. It is wise to assume that anyone may be misusing drugs, although there is a higher risk in younger people (46% of 16- to 19-year olds have used drugs at some time) and males outnumber females (by about 3:2). Many will be in active employment, although misuse is more commonly associated with poverty and unemployment. Drug availability and price are known to influence use. Previous experience may be important, as is knowledge of the desired effect to be achieved. Tightened legal consequences and sanctions go some way to controlling both supply and use. Genetic vulnerability and personality probably also contribute to risk, and the progression from use to dependence is probably determined by a combination of psychological reinforcement and pharmacogenetic factors (Farrell & Strang, 1994).

Clinical presentation

Clinical features in the workplace are seldom the signs of puncture wounds, nasal septum ulceration, respiratory depression, constipation and pupillary dilation or constriction commonly associated with drug misuse, although these may assist, together with detailed history, in assessing someone suspected of misuse. Triggers to identification include non-specific altered behaviour, with mood swings and impaired concentration; unusual aggression or irritability, resulting in poor or deteriorating relationships with colleagues, supervisors and customers; impaired performance; poor time-keeping; financial difficulties; and increased sickness absence.

Prognosis

Accurate prognosis can be difficult. The design and management of the treatment regime are important and well-structured programmes will improve outcome.

Impact on work (including effects of drugs)

In the workplace, drug misuse has both direct and indirect effects. Impairment of function from depressants potentially affects safety by reducing concentration, responsiveness to work instructions and reaction time. Similarly, a reduction in the capability for critical assessment or a reduction in cognitive function will clearly have an effect on work performance. Safety incidents may have a high human as well as financial cost and a significant adverse public reaction. Stimulants may cause elation, with loss of inhibition and reduced levels of caution in decision-making. Hallucinogenic drugs may result in intermittent impairment for many months after acute usage as a result of flashbacks. Indirectly, the need of the individual to fund the habit may create difficulties for the employer, who may find internal theft from other employees or of company assets increases.

Failure to rehabilitate may result in removal of the employee from the workplace, and the replacement of skilled and highly experienced personnel has significant operational and cost implications. Steps to prevent, or secondly to identify, treat and rehabilitate, therefore have material benefits for the employee and employer alike.

Management

Establishing policies to address the issue is a fundamental step. The company should clearly lay out its policies for prevention, treatment and support, but also the disciplinary consequences of failure to respond. This may help with self-identification or encourage referrals by colleagues or supervisors. All staff should be made aware of their responsibilities under company policy and education of personnel may be needed. The preservation of employment status remains a strong motivator in many cases, and the benefits to be achieved for the individual by intervention in the workplace should not be underestimated.

Interventions/treatment

Intervention is dependent on confirmed identification. Since the suggestive signs are far from specific, definitive confirmation may be aided by direct measurement of the drugs or their metabolites in the urine. This may be considered at pre-employment, post-incident or randomly, or as part of an after-care programme, dependent on risk assessment by the organisation.

Commitment to ensure effective treatment is essential. Acute detoxification is unlikely to be carried out in the occupational health context, but further follow-up, monitoring and maintenance of abstinence may well be effectively initiated there. The key opportunities are in terms of motivational interviewing, goal setting and referral, and early detection of relapse.

At first contact, it is important to determine whether or not employees actually accept that they have a problem with their drug use, and if so, whether they are ready or willing to do anything about it. If they are not convinced of the fact that they have a problem, or if they do not wish to change their drug use, it is unlikely that any changes will actually be made. Once a need to change is accepted, a discussion of abstinence or harm reduction as a treatment goal is the next step. In the occupational context, especially where safety is a consideration, it is likely that only the former goal will be acceptable to an employer. However, this consideration needs to be discussed carefully with employees. If they are motivated to retain employment, this improves the prospect of a good outcome. See Saunders (1994) for further discussion of a cognitive–behavioural approach to treatment.

For most occupational physicians, the main counselling or other specialist treatment interventions will be offered by another agency. It is important to become familiar with National Health Service, 'non-statutory' and other treatment facilities in the locality, and the different treatment programmes that they offer, in order that appropriate referrals can be made. Often, treatment may be on an out-patient basis, but sometimes referral for residential rehabilitation will be necessary.

Rehabilitation (implications for occupational health practice)

On completion of treatment, rehabilitation into the workplace creates challenges for all involved. Relapse rates may be high and decisions to return individuals to safety-critical positions may not be appropriate. Ongoing support in the workplace can be highly successful, where close alliances are created between the employee, the treating psychiatrist, the occupational physician and management. Progress can be monitored, success demonstrated and the employee supported. Organisations may not be able to tolerate relapses after re-entry and this is, of course, problematic for the employee. It is desirable for a post-treatment zero-tolerance policy to be openly communicated at the outset.

Prevention

Prevention ideally begins many years before employment. Attitudes are formed at an early age and success is more likely with early intervention. Charitable organisations take the message to the classroom in structured form for all ages, and the police do a sterling job in educating and influencing the views of the young. However, some educational interventions have proved counterproductive and expert advice is required in their effective planning and administration.

For employees, in-house awareness programmes are beneficial; they should cover the effects of drug misuse – both perceived positive and negative – and importantly the company's stance and policies for handling the misuse. The occupational physician would be well advised to be an active participant in the planning and implementation of a company drug policy, but should transparently leave implementation of any disciplinary requirements to line management.

Legal aspects

Employers have potential liability under both civil and criminal law to take reasonable care of the health and safety of employees and other people on their work sites (Health and Safety at Work Act etc. 1974, and Management of Health and Safety at Work Regulations 1999). In addition, there may be liabilities for the employer under the Misuse of Drugs Act 1971, should drugs of misuse be found on their premises.

References

Farrell, M. & Strang, J. (1994) Illicit drug use: aetiology, epidemiology and prevention. In *Seminars in Alcohol and Drug Misuse* (eds J. Chick & R. Cantwell), pp. 18–32. London: Gaskell.

Institute for the Study of Drug Dependence (ISDD) (1997) *Drug Misuse in Britain 1996*. London: ISDD.

Saunders, B. (1994) The cognitive–behavioural approach to the management of addictive behaviour. In *Seminars in Alcohol and Drug Misuse* (eds J. Chick & R. Cantwell), pp. 156–173. London: Gaskell.

Further reading

Faculty of Occupational Medicine (1994). *Guidelines on Testing for Drugs of Abuse in the Workplace*. London: Faculty of Occupational Medicine.

Gerada, C. & Ashworth, M. (1997) ABC of mental health. Addiction and dependence I: Illicit drugs. *British Medical Journal*, **315**, 297–300.

Health and Safety Executive (1998) *Drug Misuse at Work – A Guide for Employers*. London: HSE Books.

Rees, L., Lipsedge, M. & Ball, C. (eds) (1997) *Textbook of Psychiatry*. London: Arnold.

CHAPTER 14

Anorexia and bulimia

J. H. Lacey and N. A. Mitchell-Heggs

Introduction

Beverly Allitt, notorious child murderer, is remembered for the ghastliness of her crimes and the betrayal of her profession, and by occupational physicians, psychiatrists and those with eating disorders as having a negative effect on the employment of the latter. Allitt developed an anorexia-type illness in prison. This fact, together with mention of those with eating disorders in the investigatory Clothier Committee's report (Department of Health, 1994; see also Royal College of Nursing, 1994), resulted in the emergence of some unnecessarily over-restrictive occupational health screening practices, especially for those applying for, or already undertaking, work within the caring professions.

The chair of the Association of National Health Occupational Physicians (ANHOPs) gave evidence to the Clothier Committee. She observed that it may be difficult to assess those with personality disorder and advised that 'excessive use of counselling or medical facilities, or self-harming behaviour such as attempted suicide, self-laceration or eating disorder' may be better guides to occupational fitness than psychological testing. She suggested that applicants for nursing who show more than one of these patterns should not be accepted for nurse training 'until they have shown the ability to live an independent life, without professional support and have been in stable employment for at least two years'. The Clothier Committee endorsed this advice and felt that it would allow those going through a temporary phase of dysfunctional behaviour to stabilise. There was no suggestion in the Clothier report that all those with eating disorders were likely to mimic Allitt's behaviour; unfortunately, however, the Committee's recommendations have since been overzealously interpreted by many inexperienced occupational physicians, who have tended to apply them too rigorously, rather than relying on individual assessment and sound clinical judgement.

Eating disorders are not personality disorders and it is the latter, not the former, which should be subject to the strictures of the Committee. At times, of course, eating disorders – especially bulimia – and personality disorders may present co-morbidly, but similarly although someone with a personality disorder may develop diabetes, one would not subject all diabetics to draconian rules, especially rules which are not derived from evidence-based medicine.

Prevalence, presentation, treatment and prognosis

Anorexia and bulimia nervosa are common. Approximately 0.8% of women aged 15 to 40 years develop anorexia and 2–3% bulimia. Many more have shades of the illnesses, all of which are sub-categories of DSM–IV (American Psychiatric Association, 1994) or ICD–10 (World Health Organization, 1992). The conditions are even more common among those educational groups from which the caring professions would wish to recruit.

Bulimia nervosa occurs at normal body weight. It is manifest by binge-eating and vomiting and needs to be distinguished from the bulimic form of anorexia nervosa, where the prognosis is much worse. Bulimia nervosa develops later than anorexia, usually around 18 to 20 years of age. It occurs, unlike anorexia, in all social classes equally. It responds well to treatment: some 80% remain free of the behaviour following short treatment courses, typically weekly one-hour attendance for ten weeks, with three three-monthly follow-up appointments. Patients respond to behavioural, focal interpretative and cognitive techniques. The majority need no further medical intervention, although some 20% benefit from non-specific counselling over a further year. There is no evidence that such patients can be affected by the stresses of normal employment (as opposed to interpersonal relationships).

Anorexia nervosa is quite different. It is an often intractable condition. Treatment is usually tiered: first, out-patient support (both dietetic and psychological); then day-care or in-patient treatment. Motivated patients treated in good centres respond well, some 65% remaining clear of the disorder at follow-up. Effective treatment for adults usually involves in-patient help in specialised centres with a range of therapies – psychodynamic and cognitive – delivered individually or in groups and coupled, most importantly, with practical therapy concerning food, food preparation and lifestyle support. The move to day care has been financially driven and its efficacy compared with in-patient treatment has yet to be established. The method by which particular treatments work for the individual patient is unknown. Patients who have maintained their weight for one year and who have not engaged in any eating disorder behaviour generally do not relapse.

They may remain emotionally immature but usually compensate for this by working diligently and effectively.

Rarely, anorexia and bulimia may be an end-result of personality disorder; there are, however, many and more-common causes of disturbed eating. Anorexia and bulimia may become associated with addictive and self-damaging behaviour. This indicates a poorer prognosis unless specialised treatment is offered. At St George's in London, such a treatment programme has been available for these so-called multi-impulsives since the early 1980s. The five-year results are pleasing, with over 60% of patients who complete treatment giving up self-destructive behaviour. This group represents a small proportion of the total anorectic and bulimia population, and even among the multi-impulsive group virtually none would be considered dangerous to society.

Occupational health issues

Following publication of Clothier's report, ANHOPs issued guidance. The chair emphasised that 'Assessment of fitness must be made against the needs of the job, NOT against some pre-conceived notion of a healthy person'. She stressed that there is no need to exclude from health care training courses or employment those who have had a transitory period of psychological difficulty, provided that they have the functional capacity to carry out their work efficiently, consistently, safely and not to the detriment of others or themselves.

The caring professions in particular are enormously demanding on those who undertake them. People who are psychologically vulnerable may decompensate under the pressure; there are few predictors, but the ability to demonstrate that an individual has coped with some of the ordinary pressures of life such as study, work relationships and living away from home while not requiring intensive medical or psychological support indicates stability. It would not be necessary to refuse employment simply because an applicant was wishing, by continuing to have some counselling, to avoid the return of illness.

Not to recruit otherwise good applicants solely because of a declaration of an eating disorder would be discriminatory because, first, bulimia is virtually undetectable if an applicant wished to deny its presence, and, second, the policy would lead to general denial and discourage sufferers from seeking treatment. Further, the term 'eating disorders' is not a precise diagnosis, being too general to be linked to any particular prognosis. Each of the eating disorders is distinct in its clinical features, psychopathology, treatment needs and prognosis.

The occupational physician's assessment relies on a number of screening processes – the self-completed health questionnaire is a usual first step. The SCOFF questionnaire (Morgan *et al*, 1999; and see

> **Box 14.1** The five SCOFF questions
>
> (1) Do you make yourself *S*ick because you feel uncomfortably full?
> (2) Do you worry you have lost *C*ontrol over how much you eat?
> (3) Have you ever lost more than *O*ne stone in a three-month period?
> (4) Do you believe yourself to be *F*at when others say you are too thin?
> (5) Would you say that *F*ood dominates your life?
>
> The scale is scored as one point for every 'yes': a score of more than two indicates a likely case of anorexia or bulimia.

Box 14.1) has been shown to be effective in raising an index of suspicion in patients attending general practice and among student nurses. The five questions may be administered in written or oral form.

Some services, since Clothier, have also introduced a brief supplementary general practitioner-completed questionnaire (with specific questions about mental ill health, such as those dealing with self-harm, substance misuse and eating disorders) for those entering health care training. The experience of those using this instrument has been very positive and the information is often sufficiently comprehensive to make further medical reports unnecessary. However, those with clinically unrecognised eating disorders will obviously not be identified at this stage. Personal medical screening will still be necessary – it is at this interview that the occupational physician attempts to assess whether the problems are largely resolved or chronic. A refusal to be weighed, for example, may indicate ongoing issues.

Assessment of the severity of the eating disorder will be elicited by the history (e.g. duration, lowest weight, highest weight, use of laxatives, dietary history, amenorrhoea, etc.). Indicators of more serious psychological pathology may include self-harm, substance misuse, stealing, sexual dysfunction. A sensitive area will relate to the subjects of eating disorders who are the victims of sexual abuse. It is this group who may not, as yet, have resolved their own reactions to their life experiences but still be drawn to care for others. It is especially important to elicit through personal questioning or a medical report whether such issues have been resolved. One indicator of this may be the fact that the perpetrator has been named, parents (if not the perpetrators) and partners put in the picture, and self-blame no longer an issue. Failure to have addressed these issues may make personal work with such clients particularly painful and there may be risk of psychological decompensation, especially if good support mechanisms are not in place. Occupational clearance may be given, if the individual is considered to be psychologically robust in other respects, provided that support at times of potential stress is available.

Box 14.2 Information to seek in potential cases of eating disorder

- Length of episode(s)
- When the last episode ended
- Ongoing symptoms (self-harm, suicide attempts, substance misuse)
- Treatment
- Ongoing factors which may result in relationship difficulties
- Whether recovery is sufficiently stable to be likely to withstand the demands of the particular occupational role
- Whether the individual demonstrates an understanding of his/her own mental health to an extent which would permit helping others with similar difficulties in an objective manner and without self-detriment
- The likelihood that ongoing psychiatric support will be required, and if so, at what intensity (occasional review appointments should not cause concern, in terms of occupational fitness)

Those whose recovery from an eating disorder relies on a rigid eating timetable may find shift work and the erratic timing of meals potentially difficult. This must be discussed, anticipated and monitored if training or work includes such features. Similarly, those with unresolved attitudes to eating may be unsuited to work as dieticians.

A psychiatric report may be necessary before assessment is complete and is likely to be most informative if, in addition to confirming the history, a number of relevant specific questions are asked (Box 14.2).

Summary

Eating disorders are extremely common; the spectrum of severity is wide. While in some they may be associated with serious psychological pathology, in many it is a single entity which does not significantly affect the functions of daily activity or work.

Occupational fitness must not be decided on rigid criteria from a checklist but should be task focused – an assessment of individual fitness in relation to a specific work role.

References

American Psychiatric Association (1994) *Diagnostic and Statistical Manual of Mental Disorders* (4th edn) (DSM–IV). Washington, DC: APA.

Department of Health (1994) *The Allitt Inquiry. Independent Inquiry in Relation to Deaths and Injuries on the Children's Ward at Grantham and Kesteven General Hospital*. London: HMSO.

Morgan J. H., Reid, F. & Lacey, J. H. (1999) The SCOFF questionnaire: assessment of a new screening tool for eating disorders. *British Medical Journal*, **319**, 1467–1468.

Royal College of Nursing (1994) *The Care of Sick Children – Review of the Guidelines in the Wake of the Allitt Inquiry*. London: Royal College of Nursing.

World Health Organization (1992) *Tenth Revision of the International Classification of Diseases* (ICD–10). Geneva: WHO.

CHAPTER 15

The effects of travel on mental well-being: fear of flying and other psychiatric disorders

Su Wang and Lawrence Burns

Fast international travel is a feature of modern life. Holidaying abroad is now a common expectation. Many books and guides have been written on the physical and biological aspects of travellers' health. In contrast, little has been written on the effects of travel on mental well-being. Commercial air travel is safe and modern aircraft provide an acceptable environment for travel purposes. The number of medical in-flight incidents is small (Table 15.1).

Fear of flying

A fear of flying is common. In general, this fear is irrational and can constitute a phobic anxiety state. Recent estimates indicate that one in six adults avoid flying altogether on account of fear and only 6% of people who fly are completely free of anxiety.

If fearful flyers are able to board an aeroplane, very often they experience intense anxiety and panic during the trip, and during their holiday or business stay considerable anticipatory anxiety will almost certainly develop concerning the return journey.

Many people with a fear of flying use alcohol or medication in an attempt to relieve their intense anxiety. Straw polls of people attending fear-of-flying courses indicate that, of those who are able to fly at all, more than 50% will use alcohol or medication before a flight.

Causative factors

For people who have never flown, there may be fears about the unknown, compounded by misinformation about the aviation industry, safety factors, training of pilots and how aircraft fly. Also, a psychological process called personalisation may come into operation: some people have a tendency to take external events (especially negative ones) and apply them to themselves when there is no rational basis for doing so. Messages from the news media which may suggest that flying is unsafe

Table 15.1 Annual medical in-flight incidents recorded by one international airline (further details available from the author upon request)

	Number
Passengers	33 537 158
Incidents	3 026
Incidents related to the central nervous system (CNS)	375
Examples of CNS cases	
Anxiety	86
Drugs/alcohol	11
Unspecified psychiatric disorders	3

Fewer than a third of the CNS cases could be classified as relating to mental health.

are internalised, thereby creating anxiety and possibly avoidance behaviour. Some people who have a fear of flying may be suffering from a pre-existing panic disorder, possibly accompanied by agoraphobia; these people worry about what would happen, and how they would cope, if they were to get a panic attack while on board; unfortunately, panic attacks are more likely to arise under conditions of restriction and confinement. People with claustrophobic tendencies may also feel very uncomfortable on aeroplanes, whether small commuter ones or larger crowded ones. Other factors which may create fear include concerns about turbulence (which in reality is uncomfortable but not dangerous) and that they will fall out of the plane (i.e. that the floor of the plane will give way). Actual traumatic incidents involving accidents (such as the Manchester Airport aircraft fire of a few years ago) may result in the development of a phobic reaction.

Clinical presentation

People who have panic attacks suffer intense fear and usually have a large range of symptoms, which include increased heart rate, palpitations, trembling, disrupted patterns of breathing, light-headedness, 'butterflies' in the stomach, mental confusion, feelings of derealisation (unreality) or depersonalisation (qualitative changes within oneself) and fears of dying or losing control. There may be a fear of showing oneself up during a panic attack. Often there is hypervigilance (being selectively attuned to pick up every happening onboard the aircraft) and catastrophic thinking related to innocuous small incidents. The self-esteem or morale of fearful flyers is often poor.

Individuals with intense anxiety may, of course, show avoidance or opting-out behaviour; flights have been delayed after a panicking passenger has boarded the aircraft.

Prognosis

Provided individuals are motivated to overcome the fear of flying, the outlook is very good, assuming they receive appropriate cognitive–behavioural therapy (CBT); counselling by itself is not likely to be effective in most cases. Many people who have been grounded have overcome their fears; with appropriate assistance, the anticipatory anxiety they have experienced has turned into anticipatory pleasure.

Effect on work

An inability to fly can have serious repercussions for businesspeople whose work may involve overseas travel. Sometimes they will conceal the problem for as long as possible by sending subordinates overseas, but sooner or later the problem comes to light, often to the embarrassment of the individual concerned. Careers may be hindered by the phobia; people may avoid applying for high-level jobs which involve flying.

Management

The key issue is often to get the fearful flyer to admit to the problem. Unfortunately, some people believe that such a fear is a sign of weakness and that they would be ridiculed by their colleagues at work. Such beliefs tend to lead to a failure to address the problem unless the fear of losing one's job becomes sufficient to overcome the reluctance. If an occupational physician is approached by a sufferer, it is important to create a climate of understanding and to communicate that the individual has a recognised clinical anxiety state. Reassurance can be provided that the problem is quite common and that with appropriate clinical assistance, regardless of the aetiology, it can be overcome. Unless the occupational physician is well versed in CBT approaches, referral to a clinical psychologist, psychiatrist, or cognitive–behavioural therapist is required. It is probably best to advise the individual to refrain from flying until coping skills have been acquired in order to deal with the phobia. If it is essential that the person flies, anxiolytic medication should be considered.

Therapy

Many research studies show that CBT is the method of choice in helping people overcome panic disorder and phobic anxiety states. The cognitive part of the therapy is concerned with helping the patient think rationally (*not* positively) about the fears. Catastrophic thinking involves cognition about the worst possible outcome. As emotion (fear, etc.) can follow the (irrational) thinking, it is important that this type of thinking be challenged and become more reality based. Irrational patterns of thinking are detected and modified, thereby leading to a reduction in anxiety. The behavioural therapy may be concerned with training the person to relax deeply and the use of systematic desensitisation. Graded exposure to fear-arousing situations (visits to different parts of airports, control towers, boarding a plane, etc.), while using the newly acquired CBT coping skills, is often an essential part of the therapeutic process.

Thus, therapy has multiple components – compiling an accurate database about all aspects of flying, graded exposure to a variety of potentially fear-arousing situations and coping with anticipatory anxiety and any fear which may arise by using the cognitive and behavioural techniques.

Avia Tours runs a number of courses involving the CBT approaches, including a flight at Heathrow, Manchester, Birmingham and Glasgow Airports for people with a fear of flying. British Airways captains and cabin staff, psychologists, psychiatrists and others are involved in the courses. Details may be obtained by telephoning 01252 793 250.

Prevention

Why are so many people afraid to fly? Partly the answer lies in the frequent, often faulty and biased messages from the news media that flying is unsafe. Sometimes the news media appear to make a drama out of an incident. Such reporting can create anxiety-generating thinking in susceptible individuals – individuals who may magnify and internalise such reports. Thinking rationally about media-reported incidents involving flying or about personal experiences while flying, and having a range of anxiety-reducing coping skills are the best ways of preventing the onset of a phobic anxiety state. Where the individual has been subjected to a traumatic experience while flying, an early debriefing session with an experienced clinician may help to allay future fears.

Other psychiatric morbidity reported in association with travel

There are psychiatric conditions other than fear of flying which may be related to travel. These include:

- a mefloquine-related anxiety disorder
- schizophrenia
- affective illness
- jet lag.

Mefloquine-related anxiety disorder

Neuropsychiatric symptoms have been reported in association with the anti-malarial drug mefloquine. For specific anti-malarial advice, readers should contact specialist travel clinics or visit the MASTA website (www.masta.org).

Schizophrenia

In Jerusalem each year, some 50 tourists are admitted to hospital for psychotic episodes. This may be linked to religious delusional experiences. A study of psychiatric morbidity in Heathrow Airport found admissions for schizophrenia from the airport accounted for one-fifth of the total number of schizophrenic patients admitted to the hospital. Whether this reflects the restless mobility (*voyages pathologiques*) reported in schizophrenia is hard to tell.

Affective disorders

Abnormalities of circadian rhythm have been described in manic-depressive disorder, unipolar depression and disturbances in the sleep-wake cycle. It is not known whether these altered phase shifts in the circadian sleep–wake cycle have a role in inducing the illness or whether they are a secondary consequence of the psychiatric disorder. Noradrenaline and serotonin are implicated in depressive illness, and dopamine in mania.

Jet lag

Crossing time zones is a consequence of rapid transmeridian travel. The body clock, which adapts to a 24-hour day/night cycle, is out of synchrony with the time of the destination and requires resetting by time cues, or *Zeitgebers*, at the destination. Jet lag describes the experience of this desynchronisation. The main disruption is to the sleep–wake cycle and the person experiences fatigue, irritability, poor

Table 15.2 Estimates of how long jet lag may last

Number of time zones crossed	Number days required to adjust
Westward flights	
0–3	0
4–6	1–3
7–9	2–5
10–12	2–6
Eastward flights	
0–2	0
3–5	1–5
6–8	3–7
9–11	4–9

Box 15.1 Factors which may affect a traveller's coping capacity

(1) Type of traveller
- novice, timid, dependent traveller
- elderly

(2) Premorbid status

(3) Reasons for travel
- business travel
- social events
- family reasons
- happy events/crises.

---

concentration and may feel hungry and want to defaecate at times inappropriate to the local time. Adaptation to one to two time zones when travelling east, or one to three time zones travelling west, is probably within most people's range of adaptability. Internationally competing athletes usually require one day for every time zone crossed to regain form. Business executives with important meetings are advised to schedule these meetings several days after long flights. Table 15.2 provides estimates of how long jet lag may last.

It is interesting that sleep in patients with depression resembles sleep in normal subjects whose circadian rhythm of temperature and rapid eye movement (REM) sleep are phase advanced relative to their sleep schedule. Depression may therefore appear when travelling from east to west and hypomania when travelling from west to east.

It should be noted that the degree of disruption varies with individuals (Box 15.1) and that it tends to be more severe when travelling eastwards and the more time zones crossed.

Conclusion

Business travellers tend to be self-selected and they by and large enjoy business travel. They tend to have the travel eased for them in many ways – ticketing, check-in, baggage, fast-track facilities, restful lounge facilities, and the other benefits offered to those travelling business/ first class. They also tend to be confident travellers who, in the main, cope well with travelling. The frequent business traveller is usually cocooned by travel arrangements which deliver a sense of familiarity and security, with sufficient variation to make a trip interesting.

For the less experienced traveller, the pressures which exceed the individual's coping strategies may be encountered at any transition phase in the round trip from preparation to travel, arrival at destination, and time spent away from home to return to home.

People's lives are lived out in motifs, patterns, routines and lifestyles, which could be described as the sum functioning of coping strategies. The less robust individual may operate from a rigid and sparse store of coping strategies. Air travel consists of rapid transitions. The traveller is in unfamiliar territory and, unless an accustomed traveller, the challenges of each transition may result in decompensation, especially in someone in delicate balance. These individuals may not be able to cope with the number, diversity and rapidity of challenges at each transition experienced in the process of travel, to which must be added time zone changes, jet lag, change in climate, different culture and language, different social systems and so on experienced on arrival. Each challenge may be trivial in itself but may be daunting in the context of being in a foreign landscape of experience. For the vast majority, travel brings excitement, pleasure and new experiences. For some, the loss of moorings, being cut off from all that is familiar and secure, overwhelm their coping strategies. As more and more people travel, the travel industry may have a role in providing not only for the physical needs, but also smoother processes which recognise the emotional and psychological needs of the travelling population.

Further reading

Brown, D. (1996) *Flying Without Fear*. Oakland, CA: New Harbinger Publications.

Cook, G. C. (ed.) (1995) *Travel-Associated Disease*. London: Royal College of Physicians.

Cummings, C. T. & White, R. (1987) *Freedom From Fear of Flying*. London: Grafton Books.

Dawood, R. (1992) *Travellers' Health: How to Stay Healthy Abroad* (3rd edn). Oxford: Oxford University Press.

Moore-Ede, C., Sulzman, F. & Fuller, C. A. (1982) *The Clock That Times Us*. Cambridge, MA: Harvard University Press.

Swanson, V., McIntosh, I. & Power, K. (1998) Flight related anxieties and health problems. *Travel Medicine International*, 16, 83–86.

Waterhouse, J. M., Minors, D. S. & Waterhouse, M. E. (1990) *Your Body Clock: How to Live With It, Not Against It*. Oxford: Oxford University Press.

Yaffe, M. (1992) *Taking the Fear Out of Flying*. London: David & Charles.

CHAPTER 16

Critical incidents and violence at work

Ian Palmer and Charles Baron

Introduction

Although anyone may be the victim of threatened or actual violence at work, certain occupations carry a higher risk of this. This is particularly true of those dealing with people who are potentially more violent. Police officers, probation staff, prison officers and social workers may all fall into this category of occupation, but staff in the health care, teaching, retail and banking sectors, as well as those representing authority, have all been shown to be at risk, for a variety of different reasons.

Violence against one's person is a particularly difficult form of trauma, which may give rise to stress reactions. Other types of critical or traumatic incident, not involving violence but where there is a serious threat to the safety either of the individual or of some third party, where the threat or actual harm is witnessed, may also be psychologically distressing. These are less easy to predict and can arise from major human disasters such as the fires at Hillsborough stadium and King's Cross railway station. Certain occupations, however, may be at greater risk of experiencing or witnessing such incidents and these will generally include those in the emergency services and the armed forces.

Most individuals cope well under adversity. It is a mistake to overestimate the numbers who will react poorly to a critical incident and it is incorrect to assume that most people will be 'traumatised' by such events. All will, however, be changed by their experiences, and not infrequently for the better. It is important to avoid giving medical labels to normal reactions but it is equally important not to miss any post-trauma mental illness. Although distress and post-traumatic symptoms are common after exposure to traumatic events, most cases settle without professional intervention. However, some may lead to full-blown post-traumatic mental disorders, including post-traumatic stress disorder (PTSD).

Stress reactions

Acute stress reactions

These are psychological reactions which occur during the critical incident. They may range from blind panic, fear or agitation, through to withdrawal, stupor and so on. These symptoms may be seen in the minority of individuals. The worse the critical incident is, the more likely they are to occur, but they settle rapidly when the stimulus is removed.

Post-traumatic stress reactions

Post-traumatic stress reactions are quite common and may be erroneously diagnosed as PTSD. The symptoms are similar, varying only in degree, duration and context – they are re-experiencing, avoidance and arousal phenomena, with their associated behaviours.

- *Re-experiencing* – recurrent, unwanted, intrusive thoughts, images, sounds, smells; 'triggers' cause distress and physical arousal; it may include nightmares, 'as if' phenomena or 'flashbacks'.
- *Avoidance* – avoiding thoughts and things associated with the event; feeling emotionally isolated; loss of interest in things previously enjoyed.
- *Arousal* – feeling 'on edge', unable to relax; irritable and aggressive; difficulty in sleeping and concentrating; forgetfulness.
- *Associated behaviours* – substance misuse, especially excessive intake of alcohol; relationship problems; risk-taking activities; impulsiveness; survivor guilt; depression.

These reactions usually settle within 6 to 12 weeks but are problematic for some individuals, as is grief. Indeed, grief is a good simile because post-trauma psychological processes are like the mourning process through which we all go and with which a few have problems.

Post-trauma mental illness

Post-traumatic stress disorder is not synonymous with post-trauma mental illness and should be diagnosed only following expert assessment, when an individual has been exposed to exceptionally life-threatening events and the symptoms interfere significantly in numerous areas of that person's life.

Post-trauma mental illness may reveal itself in many ways and at varying times after an incident. Those closest to the individual will be the first to notice any change, as relationship problems are common. If work is suffering it is important for colleagues and management to encourage individuals to seek help.

Prevention

Employers can take action to reduce the risks of violence to their staff. They can also minimise the risk of serious (life-threatening) harm to employees from accidents. Critical incidents, however, are not preventable (fire-fighters attend fires in which children may die and soldiers are paid to fight and possibly see their friends and colleagues killed). Nonetheless, it may be possible for an employer to plan for critical incidents and ensure that actions are taken to reduce the risk of psychological harm arising from them.

Assessing risks

The Management of Health and Safety at Work Regulations 1999 require that employers assess the risks to their employees and take action to minimise those risks by effective planning, organisation, control, monitoring and review. It is a good idea for employers to have a policy relating to managing violence at work and this may either be a stand-alone policy or part of a wider-ranging health and safety policy.

A good way of assessing risks of violence to staff is to ask them about situations where they have felt threatened. A questionnaire survey might help with this. Encouraging staff to report all actual and potential violent incidents through an effective reporting system and analysing the results of these reports are also essential. By using the results from such reports, as well as their knowledge of a job, good managers can predict who is at greatest risk, where, when, how and, most important, why.

Minimising risks

There will be many things which an employer can do to minimise risks. These in themselves will give employees more confidence about their personal safety and reduce anxieties associated with perceived risks. The list below is by no means exhaustive.

(1) Work systems:
- identifying and communicating about known violent 'customers'
- logging staff movements
- ringing in
- two-person (or more) activities
- minimising cash movements
- checking credentials of clients
- arrangements for safe parking/travel

(2) The environment:
- provision of good seating, lighting and information in waiting areas
- video-cameras

- personal attack alarms
- coded security locks
- glass panels for better visibility of colleagues
- security screens at counters

(3) Training and information:
- recognising and defusing aggression
- using safe systems of work
- using safety equipment
- self-defence (in some situations).

Some of these measures may have an undesired effect. For example, security screens may make it more difficult to communicate, and thus increase tension and make aggression more likely.

Planning for critical incidents

In order to facilitate post-traumatic interventions, it is necessary to ensure that managers and the work group are properly educated and informed about:

- recognising critical incidents
- recognising stress reactions
- providing appropriate support.

Initiating support processes and reminding staff about access to professional help (from the occupational health department or counselling services) are facilitated by defining a critical incident in advance so that all staff know when one has occurred. For example, components of a definition for a fire crew might include:

- multiple fatalities or life-threatening injuries
- where the victim is a colleague or otherwise known to the fire crew
- where the victim is a child
- where fire crew feel that they are partly to blame for a fatality (too slow, wrong action).

Post-trauma interventions

Stress reactions are an interaction between the individual, the event and that person's psychosocial environment. Psychological 'protection' is afforded by adaptive coping and psychological defence mechanisms. These will be facilitated by previous exposure and mastery of similar events, intelligence and cognitive abilities, and the desire to learn from situations. Groups can also protect an individual by instilling a unity of purpose, loyalty, mutual kinship and a group ethos, making employees feel supported and valued.

Psychological debriefing has not been shown to prevent post-traumatic mental disorders or illness. Recent evidence indicates that early, single interventions may be actively harmful and cannot therefore be recommended. Any intervention should be as simple and humane as possible.

Immediate

- Show human kindness.
- Maintain normality and if possible keep the person at work.
- Encourage group support and encourage talking.
- Reinforce the normality of the reactions.
- Prepare a quick run-through of what happened.
- Managers should lead by example and get involved appropriately from the outset.
- Offer open access to help – give contact numbers.

Short term

- Keep the person at work or ensure earliest possible return to work.
- Encourage the group to 'look after its own'.
- Allow the individual to choose when (and whether) any formal intervention is wanted and time it accordingly.
- Analyse what happened, involve the individual(s) and learn the lessons – enshrine them in protocols and training by using the episode to reinforce the teaching received.
- Management should be involved where appropriate.
- Show other staff that the organisation cares and looks after its staff.

Medium/long term

- Look for change in personality, work patterns or efficiency.
- Note sickness absences after the incident.
- Do not be afraid to ask whether the individual is all right.
- Expect others' interest to wane, while accepting that the individual may still be suffering.
- Offer access to formal psychiatric or psychological assessment if the individual requests it, if there are problems from the outset or if the reactions do not settle after 6 to 12 weeks.

Treatments and prognosis

Assessment should be early and look for treatable mental illness. Depression should be treated vigorously. Cognitive, behavioural and imaginal techniques (such as eye movement desensitisation and reprocessing – EMDR) are useful therapeutic tools. They are of proven benefit with certain problems but they are not panaceas. The therapy must be tailored to the individual's needs; the main benefit will be in helping people to gain mastery over their intrusive thoughts and avoidance behaviours, and in coming to terms with the change wrought by the trauma so that they may get on with their life once more (a similar process to grief work).

Interventions work well but the genesis of post-trauma mental illness is complex and some individuals will require in-depth or long-term help – they will be the minority.

Further reading

Health and Safety Executive (1997) *Violence at Work: A Guide for Employers*. London: HSE Books.

Hobbs, M., Mayou, R., Harrison, B., *et al* (1996) A randomised controlled trial of psychological debriefing for victims of road traffic accidents. *British Medical Journal*, **313**, 1438–1439.

O'Brien, L. S. (1998) *Traumatic Events and Mental Health*. Cambridge: Cambridge University Press.

CHAPTER 17

Chronic fatigue syndrome

Michael Sharpe and Derek White

The condition

Chronic fatigue syndrome (CFS), post-viral fatigue syndrome (PVFS), neurasthenia and myalgic encephalomyelitis (ME) are terms used to describe an idiopathic syndrome of chronic fatigue and disability. The nature, pathology and aetiology of this syndrome remain controversial and the descriptive term chronic fatigue syndrome (CFS) is preferred. The core aspects of case definition are shown in Box 17.1.

Causative factors

There is no established single cause. Multiple causes must therefore be considered. These may be classified as biological, psychological and social, and then further divided into predisposing, precipitating and perpetuating factors (see Table 17.1).

Biological factors

These are not fully understood. Patients commonly describe their illness as beginning with flu-like symptoms. Although a short period of

---

Box 17.1 Core aspects of case definition of chronic fatigue syndrome

- Clinically evaluated medically unexplained fatigue of at least six months' duration that leads to a substantial reduction in previous level of activities.
- Some definitions require additional symptoms, including: subjective memory impairment, sore throat, tender lymph nodes, muscle pain, joint pain, headache, unrefreshing sleep, post-exertional malaise lasting more than 24 hours.
- Patients with certain psychiatric syndromes, including psychosis, severe depression, substance misuse and eating disorders, are excluded.

Table 17.1 A hypothetical causal model of CFS

Type of cause	Examples of causative factors		
	Predisposing	Precipitating	Perpetuating
Biological	Genetic pre-disposition (?)	Virus infection	Consequences of inactivity Sleep disturbance (?) Immune disturbance (?) Neuroendocrine disturbance (?)
Psychological	Vulnerable personality (?) Previous depression	Psychological response to stress	Attribution of symptoms to disease Fear of making symptoms worse Coping by avoidance
Social	Stigma of psychiatric illness	Stress	Personal conflicts Iatrogenic factors Occupational factors

fatigue and exhaustion is common after flu, glandular fever and similar illnesses, fatigue lasting longer than six months is not readily attributable to viral infection. Physical deconditioning from inactivity, somatic manifestations of depression and anxiety, and sleep disturbance may all contribute.

Psychological factors

Although there is a strong association with depression and anxiety disorders, these do not offer a full explanation of the illness in most cases. Patients may believe that symptoms indicate organic disease and fear activity-induced exacerbation. The resulting avoidance of activity may cause severe disability.

Social factors

Patients may emphasise physical rather than emotional symptoms because of social stigma. Misleading information may reinforce this 'medical' bias. Conflicts over life direction, chronic stress and work dissatisfaction are often important.

Clinical presentation

Mental and physical fatigue exacerbated by activity is the central symptom. Patients often report being able to perform for brief periods, but that they subsequently experience severe fatigue for periods of hours or days thereafter. Other symptoms include muscle pain, dizziness and breathlessness, unrefreshing sleep, tender lymph glands and symptoms of irritable bowel syndrome. Physical examination is typically unremarkable, and the definite physical signs require an alternative explanation. In the workplace, cases often come to notice as a single long absence, but can be found among those with frequent short absences where the individual is seeking to maintain attendance.

Prognosis

The prognosis for full recovery is good for patients seen in general practice but poor in those with chronic fatigue syndrome severe enough for hospital referral. It is also worse for patients who have a conviction that the cause of the illness is purely 'physical'. Clinical experience also suggests that poor social and occupational functioning before the onset of illness predicts poor outcome. Pre-illness dissatisfaction with employment seems to reduce the chances of a return to work.

Effect on work

Patients may struggle to perform to their usual standard or may have recurrent or prolonged sick leave. Uncertainty about the diagnosis may lead to friction with employers and colleagues, who tend to lose sympathy over the length of absence.

Assessment

Medical and psychiatric assessments are recommended in every case.

Excluding organic disease

A few patients will be found to have occult organic disease. However, if a careful history and physical examination do not point to alternative diagnoses, laboratory investigation will add little.

Identifying psychiatric syndromes

All patients should have a psychiatric history taken and mental state examination, in order to detect evidence of major depression, anxiety and panic disorder. Suicidal intent should also be evaluated. A smiling presentation is a common reason to miss depression.

Wider assessment

It is desirable to make a systematic assessment of possible and reversible perpetuating factors in each case. This should include the individual's beliefs about the illness, coping behaviour, emotional state, physiological condition and interpersonal and occupational problems (Table 17.1).

Treatment and rehabilitation

General treatment should include acknowledgement of the reality of the patient's symptoms, the provision of accurate medical information (avoiding unproductive argument) and encouragement of a gradual return to normal activities. Further treatment is summarised in Box 17.2.

Prevention

Given that we do not know the cause of CFS, prevention is difficult. Screening at the point of recruitment for current or partially recovered CFS or depression may identify vulnerability. Stress may be a factor.

Box 17.2 Summary of the treatment approaches for CFS

Pharmacological
Consider antidepressant drugs.
Avoid polypharmacy.

Non-pharmacological
Gradual increase in exercise.
Cognitive–behavioural therapy.
Work rehabilitation.

Pharmacological treatments
Many pharmacological treatments have been suggested for patients with CFS but none has proven efficacy. There is some evidence to support the use of antidepressant drugs.

Exercise therapy
This should be considered for patients who are physically inactive. With appropriate supervision a graded increase in physical activity is helpful in improving function and relieving symptoms. The simplistic application of exercise regimens is unlikely to be helpful, however.

Psychotherapy
Although brief psychotherapeutic approaches may have a place, the only psychological treatment for CFS supported by evidence is cognitive–behavioural therapy (CBT). CBT is especially well suited to helping patients achieve a more positive view of the illness and adopt more effective coping strategies. Randomised trials of rehabilitative CBT have demonstrated its effectiveness compared with conservative approaches. CBT places particular emphasis on helping patients to reappraise their illness beliefs, increasing activity and solving social problems. A typical course comprises 10 to 20 weekly individual treatment sessions.

Anecdotal evidence suggests that the uncomplaining employee who becomes overloaded may be at risk.

Legal issues

The Disability Discrimination Act has significant implications for many aspects of the employment of those with CFS.

Occupational rehabilitation

The management in the workplace of employees suffering from CFS can be difficult for all concerned. A carefully planned and supervised programme of workplace rehabilitation may be helpful where both patient and employer are willing to try it. Coordination with other treatment and rehabilitation measures (e.g. CBT) is important. Work rehabilitation will usually need to start with dramatically reduced workload and hours of work that are gradually increased depending on progress. It can be a lengthy process and the success rate is moderate at best. Lack of, or refusal to accept, appropriate treatment by the National Health Service and misleading advice are common problems. Employers, particularly those in the more competitive sectors, can seldom wait sufficiently long for recovery and, consequently, termination of employment may have to be considered. The occupational physician may be asked also to advise on retirement on grounds of ill health, for which a common criterion is permanent inability to undertake normal duties – a requirement unlikely to be satisfied unless the incapacity is of long duration and unresponsive to treatment. Against this background the occupational physician can have an important role in supporting both patient and employer, working towards an optimal outcome and helping prevent ongoing difficulties which are not in the long-term interests of either.

Further reading

Campling, F. & Sharpe, M. (2002) *Chronic Fatigue Syndrome (CFS/ME): The Facts* (A self-help guide). Oxford: Oxford University Press.

Joint Working Party of the Royal Colleges of Physicians, Psychiatrists and General Practitioners (1996) *Chronic Fatigue Syndrome*. London: Royal College of Physicians.

Mounstephen, A. & Sharpe, M. (1997) Chronic fatigue syndrome and occupational health. *Occupational Medicine*, **47**, 217–227.

Sharpe, M., Chalder, T., Palmer, I., *et al* (1997) Chronic fatigue syndrome. A practical guide to assessment and management. *General Hospital Psychiatry*, **19**, 185–199.

Wessely, S., Hotopf, M. H. & Sharpe, M. (1998) *Chronic Fatigue and Its Syndromes*. Oxford: Oxford University Press.

CHAPTER 18

Schizophrenia and delusional disorders

Trevor Turner and Paul Litchfield

Introduction

Schizophrenia and delusional disorders are forms of psychosis, that is to say, severe mental illnesses in which the sufferer loses contact with reality because of the symptoms experienced. The lifetime prevalence is about 1% in any population. Early symptoms are easily missed and tend to pre-date diagnosis by up to several years. Presentations vary, depending on age, family background, culture and ethnicity, and level of education. There is no diagnostic test but the clinical diagnosis has high reliability.

Causative factors

The current model is neurodevelopmental, with a considerable genetic basis. A number of genes seem to contribute to the morbidity risk; thus, 10% of the first-degree relatives of a person suffering from schizophrenia will probably likewise suffer, as will 50% of the offspring of two parents with schizophrenia. Both *in utero* and perinatal trauma to the brain seem to enhance the likelihood of illness. Enlarged ventricles, and damage to the frontal and temporal lobes, are common findings from computerised tomography, magnetic resonance imaging or positron emission tomography brain scans.

Clinical presentation

The symptoms of schizophrenia are commonly divided into the positive and the negative (Table 18.1). The former are quickly recognised, leading as they do to strange behaviours and impaired social functioning. Most common are the 'voices' (auditory hallucinations), which seem to be absolutely real, that comment on or order the sufferer's behaviour, and come and go at random. These may be accompanied by an impaired pattern of thinking ('formal thought disorder'), which makes it difficult for patients to explain their experiences or activities. Repeated thought

Table 18.1 The key symptoms of schizophrenia

Positive symptoms	Negative symptoms
Hallucinations (especially voices referring to the sufferer in the third person or giving running commentary) Delusions Passivity experience Thought disorder/interference	Flat affect Social withdrawal Poverty of speech Lack of drive/motivation Anhedonia

block, whereby one's mind seems to go blank and empty constantly, may occur alongside the sense of one's thoughts being inserted from outside or taken away, and the distressing feeling that other people know what you are thinking and can somehow read your thoughts. Passivity experience, a symptom often underdiagnosed, describes the sense of not being in control of one's behaviour, thoughts or feelings. All of this may relate to the formation of delusions, or complex delusional systems, namely false beliefs, unshakeable by argument, that one is being plotted against, controlled, mocked, or even that one has special powers.

More insidious are the negative symptoms, of impaired concentration and social withdrawal. Flattened affect and alogia (inability to think) are characteristic, and they lead to self-neglect, poverty of speech and a lack of drive or interest in things generally. Difficulty in concentrating or organising one's life may be the social presentation.

Although schizophrenia is a disorder usually presenting in the late teens or twenties, impairing personality development and skills, and in particular the ability to obtain qualifications, delusional disorders have a mean age of onset between 40 and 55 years. Furthermore, sufferers will have no obvious abnormality in terms of the way they speak or their public behaviour: they will simply have one or more delusional beliefs about, for example, things being done to them. Although delusions often are paranoid (that is to say, things around them have a special significance, and the coincidental becomes significant), they may not always be persecutory. Delusions can include a conviction of illness, morbid jealousy, a sense of being defrauded (which can lead to many legal actions being taken) or a belief that other people are interfering with their work in various ways. Thus the superficial presentation may be of depression or anxiety, and the insidious onset is often missed.

Prognosis

Prognosis will depend on age of onset (the later the better), insight, response to treatment and the presence of negative symptoms. The best outcomes occur when diagnosis is made within weeks of symptoms beginning, positive symptoms are eliminated by medication and there is good family support. A presentation of mostly negative symptoms, over a number of years, in someone of poor family background and limited abilities, would indicate prolonged disability. Nearly 20% of patients with schizophrenia make a full recovery, up to 30% need continuing high-dependence care and the remaining 50% have varying levels of independence, a number being able to work at least part time. Over half of patients, however, are non-compliant with medication; illicit drug use is not uncommon, and anti-psychiatry stigma compromises insight and family support.

Delusional disorders can respond well to medication provided patients have the insight to accept it, but this often occurs only after a number of relapses.

Effect on work

Schizophrenia has a profound effect on one's ability to think, to concentrate, to relate to other people and to organise oneself. Positive symptoms cause the greatest problems at work; for example, they often lead to embarrassing outbursts or bizarre allegations, sometimes relating to colleagues. Other members of staff may become alarmed and concerned for their own safety, even though episodes of violence at work are rare. Negative symptoms have a more general adverse effect on performance and attendance, and sufferers may come to the attention of occupational health staff through normal management referrals. Of all mental health problems, schizophrenia probably has the greatest residual stigma and sufferers often deny their condition at recruitment and thereafter.

Continuing symptom relief requires medication, yet typical side-effects of antipsychotics include sedation, parkinsonism (particularly tremor and facial immobility) and a sense of demotivation. Particular problems are likely to arise if the individual is required to drive, operate heavy machinery or undertake tasks where fine manual dexterity is required. Many patients experience an inner restlessness, with akathisia (inability to sit still) as its outward presentation; this only rarely causes functional employment problems but can cause difficulties if the individual fulfils a role where interpersonal contact with customers is important.

Management

The first step in the management of someone who seemingly has schizophrenia or a delusional disorder is to exclude the rare organic causes of psychosis, such as hypothyroidism, Wilson's disease and systemic lupus erythematosus.

Most employees with schizophrenia come to the attention of occupational health staff during health screening at recruitment. The assessment process is the same as for any chronic disability and should consist of determining functional capability for the post, identifying barriers to effective performance and defining adjustments which may overcome the disability. In general, individuals with schizophrenia fare best if placed in a controlled environment, where demands are more constant than variable, and pressures such as deadlines or confrontation are minimised. The chronicity and the severity of the condition will have a significant effect on precise capabilities, but most sufferers who successfully remain in employment do so at a level below that which might seem appropriate to their intellect or academic achievement.

It is unusual for people with schizophrenia to hold management positions successfully, and positions where close teamwork is essential can also be difficult. Long-term employment is more likely to be associated with a well-defined set of duties which can be discharged with minimal interaction with others. Occupational histories often chart a drift down from high expectations to menial employment because inadequate attention is paid to appropriate placement. For the more severely affected, supported placement schemes can be helpful in introducing an individual with schizophrenia back into work.

Treatment and rehabilitation

Medication is the mainstay of continuing psychological and social stability. The standard drugs, such as chlorpromazine or haloperidol, are dopamine blockers, and so have the side-effects of sedation and movement disorders. Anticholinergics can be of benefit, but sexual problems and drowsiness further impair compliance. Fortunately, a number of newer, 'atypical' antipsychotics are now available, with increased acceptability, and even effectiveness with previously treatment-resistant conditions. These include clozapine, risperidone, olanzapine and quetiapine, effective primarily via serotonin receptors, and thus they rarely cause parkinsonism.

Effective communication is as important in an occupational context as it is in a social one. Patients require careful counselling about suitable forms of employment and the management of expectations is critical. Potential employers and colleagues may require considerable reassurance when considering the employment of an individual with schizophrenia and the accounts of the disease published in fiction and the popular press are often unhelpful. Development of a mental health policy for the organisation can be an effective means of addressing the educational challenges which exist in the workplace with regard to this condition. Management of an acute psychotic episode at work requires tact and calm perseverance. Withdrawal of the individual from the workplace is the first priority but should be conducted while attempting to reassure management and colleagues, who are likely themselves to be emotionally charged and quite possibly frightened. Early liaison with the individual's own general practitioner or psychiatrist (or community keyworker) is mandatory and every effort should be made to discharge the patient into appropriate care.

Reintroducing an employee back into work after an acute psychotic episode, especially if this manifested at work, requires care and patience. Education of others in the workplace about the condition, within the constraints of confidentiality, is critical, but damage to working relationships, especially where paranoia has been a dominant feature, can be irreparable. Adjustment of duties, as outlined above, is an important feature of successful rehabilitation and a temporary reduction in hours to ease the individual back into the discipline of work can be helpful. If redeployment is essential, either because suitable adjustments cannot be made in the former work area or because of damage to relationships, then education remains critical and the new management should be helped to understand that the individual may well be slow in terms of picking up new skills, as a function of the illness, even though intellectual capability may be unimpaired.

Prevention

Controlling occupational pressures can help to reduce the risk of relapse and the early signs of relapse may first become apparent at work. Occupational physicians should maintain regular contact with an employee who has schizophrenia, as for someone with any other chronic medical problem, and management should be alerted to the early signs of deterioration so that the assistance of occupational health staff can be enlisted as soon as is practicable.

Legal aspects

Individuals with schizophrenia will normally fall within the scope of the Disability Discrimination Act and their cases should be handled with this in mind at every stage in employment, from recruitment through attendance and performance problems to retirement. Making adjustments for those with mental health problems can be harder for management to conceptualise and occupational health staff have a key role in explaining what can be done and in encouraging compliance while maintaining an objective view of what is practical.

The health and safety of other staff or the public is often cited as a concern by management when employing someone with schizophrenia. Making an assessment, with the help of hospital and primary care colleagues, of the likelihood of violent behaviour is critical and in most cases appropriate reassurance can be given. Special consideration needs to be given for posts where the individual has responsibility for the vulnerable members of society and a higher threshold for acceptance would be applied.

Further reading

Drug and Therapeutics Bulletin (1995) The drug treatment of patients with schizophrenia. *Drug and Therapeutics Bulletin*, **33** (11), 81–86.

Mason, P., Harrison, G., Glazebrook, C., *et al* (1995) Characteristics of outcome in schizophrenia at 13 years. *British Journal of Psychiatry*, **167**, 596–603.

Thomas, C. S. & Lewis, S. (1998) Which atypical antipsychotic? *British Journal of Psychiatry*, **172**, 106–109.

Turner, T. H. (1997) ABC of mental health. Schizophrenia. *British Medical Journal*, **315**, 108–111.

Wilkinson, G. & Kendrick, T. (1996) *A Carer's Guide to Schizophrenia*. London: Royal Society of Medicine Press.

CHAPTER 19

Organic states

Chris Ball and Alan Scott

Introduction

Organic psychiatric disorders are those in which examination and investigation will uncover some cerebral or systemic pathology which are responsible for, or contributing to, the mental condition (Lishman, 1998). The commonest of these are the dementing disorders (e.g. Alzheimer's disease) or delirium, which tend to be associated with later life. As the age structure of the population changes we may see more elderly people working and these problems will become more of an issue. In the workplace, however, these problems are at present still relatively rare. It is not clear to what extent organic problems affect the workforce but certain professions have a long history of problems (e.g. mercury poisoning in hatters).

A number of symptoms and signs should alert occupational physicians to the fact that changes in the productivity, time keeping and effectiveness of the workers under their care are due to organic problems and we will take these in turn.

'Neurotic' symptoms

Anxiety, depression and psychosomatic complaints are common but non-specific symptoms. They will often pre-date overt cognitive symptoms. Disorders of the temporal lobe commonly present in this way, as do many types of poisoning (e.g. lead, mercury).

Attention and concentration

The ability to attend to a task in a sustained way is vital for its completion. Subtle defects may be difficult to demonstrate clinically. An inability to concentrate is a common, early and non-specific symptom of organic disorders.

Fatigue

Fatigue is difficult to define but may be both mental and physical. The status of chronic fatigue syndrome as an organic or functional disorder remains ambiguous (see Chapter 17). Illnesses which are difficult to diagnose early (e.g. multiple sclerosis, Parkinson's disease) may present with fatigue. The common causes of fatigue are:

* depression
* drugs (beta-blockers, diuretics, hypnotics)
* alcohol
* Parkinson's disease
* multiple sclerosis
* post-concussional syndromes
* endocrine disorders
* exposure to chemicals such as lead, solvents, carbon monoxide.

Memory

Memory problems are often the earliest signs of an organic disorder. It is usually hard to date the onset of such problems; in retrospect it is usually possible to see that they have been present for some time. Occasionally they present acutely (e.g. in Korsakov's syndrome and cases of carbon monoxide poisoning). The common causes of memory dysfunction are:

* dementia (Alzheimer's disease, vascular disease, HIV infection, poisoning with a heavy metal)
* Korsakov's syndrome
* thyroid dysfunction
* drugs (tricyclic antidepressants, benzodiazepines)
* head injury.

Frontal lobe symptoms

Although they have been called the 'silent areas' of the brain, the frontal lobes are involved in high-level cognitive tasks vital for many occupations. The symptoms of damage to the frontal lobes include:

* decreased intellectual drive and apathy
* personality change
* irritability and tactlessness
* euphoria
* concrete thinking and perseveration.

The causes of such symptoms are typically:

* head injury
* tumour

- syphilis
- multiple sclerosis
- poisoning with mercury, manganese or carbon disulphide.

Parietal lobe symptoms

The parietal lobes are important in the recognition and manipulation of objects in space, including the person's own body. Thus the symptoms of damage to these lobes include:

- apraxia (difficulty manipulating objects)
- agnosia (difficulty in recognising objects)
- topographical disorientation
- disturbances of body image or neglect
- cortical sensory loss.

The common causes of parietal lobe damage are:

- dementia (Alzheimer's disease)
- vascular lesions
- tumours
- head injury.

Temporal lobe symptoms

Lesions of the temporal lobe are rarely silent. Psychiatric symptoms, both neurotic and psychotic, are common, as are memory problems. They include:

- amnesia
- hallucinations and delusions
- depression and anxiety
- sensory dysphasia.

Causes of damage to the temporal lobes include:

- dementias
- vascular lesions
- trauma
- tumours
- encephalitis
- multiple sclerosis
- poisoning with organic lead or bromomethane.

Assessing organic states

Identifying a disorder as 'organic' can be difficult. The mental state may mimic a 'functional' disorder very closely (see Table 19.1). A high index

Table 19.1 Organic *v.* functional psychiatric problems

	Organic	Functional
Onset	Slow onset	Clear-cut onset
Memory problems	Present	Usually absent
Past psychiatric history	Unlikely	Likely
Physical examination	Signs commonly present	Signs unlikely
Investigations	Abnormalities	No abnormalities
Answers to questions	Attempts to answer/confabulation	'Don't know'

of suspicion must always be maintained. (For further details of assessment, see Rees *et al*, 1997.)

History

The presenting problems of a person with an organic disorder are likely to include some of the following:

- poor productivity
- poor time keeping
- neurotic symptoms
- memory disturbance
- change of behaviour (withdrawal, apathy, decreased self-care)
- abnormal behaviour (urinating inappropriately, violence).

The history of the presenting problems is one of slow change; it is often hard to say when they started. The person may have little insight into the problems and taking a co-lateral history from those at work and at home is vital. The difficulties may well have been seen earlier at home, where there are not the routines of work. Organic disorders due to chemicals, however, can present acutely.

The issues to explore when taking the patient's history, in an overall systematic enquiry, are as follows:

- presenting complaint
- changes in activities and behaviour (e.g. hobbies)
- past medical history
- drug and alcohol history.

Physical examination

A detailed physical examination is required. The neurological signs that accompany organic cerebral disorders may be subtle (e.g. visual field defects, dysgraphaesthesia) and must be assiduously sought, as must signs of systemic disease (e.g. clubbing, heart murmurs).

Mental state examination

The presence of any form of cognitive impairment should alert the examiner to the presence of an organic disorder. Routine 'bedside' tests such as the Abbreviated Mental Test Score are unlikely to prove sensitive to subtle changes. As a minimum, the Mini-Mental State Examination (MMSE; Folstein *et al*, 1975) should be performed. If the examiner suspects cognitive problems from clues in the history (e.g. gaps, vagueness, unclear thinking), then a detailed assessment from a psychologist should be sought.

Investigation

Standard haematological investigations may reveal some abnormalities (hypothyroidism, diabetes). Where indicated, more specialist tests of blood (e.g. for mercury or methaemoglobin) or urine (e.g. for lead) should be carried out. To reach a diagnosis, imaging (computerised tomography or magnetic resonance imaging) or functional tests (electro-encephalography, single photon emission computerised tomography) may have to be performed.

Anyone under the age of 65 with suspected dementia should be referred for investigation to a specialist such as a psychiatrist or neurologist.

Managing organic states

Managing organic states in the workplace is difficult. If a clearly defined underlying cause for the problem can be found and this remedied within a short time (e.g. hypothyroidism), then the person is likely to be able to resume the previous level of employment. If there is a prolonged illness or exposure to a toxin (e.g. manganese) it is unlikely that the person will return to the premorbid level of functioning, even if the underlying cause is remedied or removed.

For routine work requiring little in the way of decision-making or flexibility, tasks may be undertaken with quite profound levels of impairment yet managed well. Tasks that require little flexibility or complex activity but are 'safety critical' (e.g. look-out for a track repair gang) should not be undertaken by those with poor concentration.

Performance on tasks requiring complex, higher-level functioning is more likely to be impaired by subtle changes in cognitive state, although persons with such disability may be able to manage day-to-day living at a high level (e.g. an accountant who could no longer manage company finances could complete the *Daily Mail* crossword, having previously managed *The Times* crossword). Detailed cognitive assessment will give indications as to the kinds of problem an individual is likely to experience.

Occupational therapy assessments using instruments such as the Assessment of Motor and Process Skills (AMPS; Fisher, 2001) give information on an individual's ability to plan and execute complex motor tasks. Information from these is useful when considering the type of work someone might be capable of performing and in the planning of a rehabilitation package.

In summary, then, the management of organic states in the workplace involves the following steps:

- identify and rectify (if possible) the underlying cause
- identify the residual cognitive deficits
- identify motor and processing abnormalities
- match these to the demands of the work tasks and environment
- evaluate the safety considerations – these are paramount.

Conclusions

It is not known what effects organic psychiatric disorders have in the workplace. They have recently had a high media profile (e.g. new-variant Creutzfeld–Jacob disease) despite their relatively low prevalence in those of working age. The financial and personal implications of organic states are, however, very great and all doctors must maintain a high level of suspicion that the psychiatric syndrome they are seeing has an underlying 'organic' basis; if there is one, its cause must be identified. They must also be aware of the impact that these disorders are having in the person's workplace and act accordingly.

References

Fisher, A. G. (2001) *AMPS: Assessment of Motor and Process Skills* (4th edn). Fort Collins, CO: Three Star Press.

Folstein, M. S., Folstein, S. A. & McHugh, P. R. (1975) Mini-Mental State. A practical method for grading the cognitive state for the clinician. *Journal of Psychiatric Research*, **12**, 189–198.

Lishman, W. A. (1998) *Organic Psychiatry* (3rd edn). Oxford: Blackwell.

Rees, L., Lipsedge, M. S. & Ball, C. J. (1997) *Textbook of Psychiatry*. London: Arnold.

CHAPTER 20

Personality disorders in the workplace

Alison Martin, Maurice Lipsedge and James Watson

Definition

Descriptions of personality refer to 'what sort of person this is'; an individual's personality is like a coin the sides of which are the individual's self-view and other people's views of him or her. Personality is the sum of relatively enduring dispositions and habitual behaviour patterns, that is the *traits* which together form the individual's personality structure. Genetic and environmental factors influence this. Traits contrast with *states*, which are relatively short-term conditions that include a range of normal reactions to events and stimuli. States which clearly represent variations from normal constitute *illnesses*. Traits are present to a greater or lesser extent in everyone; disorders of personality occur when they are present or absent to an extreme degree.

Eight specific disorders are listed in ICD–10 (World Health Organization, 1992):

- paranoid
- schizoid
- antisocial
- emotionally unstable
- histrionic
- anankastic (obsessional)
- anxious
- dependent.

All of these involve problems with emotion, interpersonal relationships and self-control, and thus have an impact on adaptation to working environments. The greater the personality difficulties, the greater are the chances of poor functioning in the workplace.

Presentation of problems

At work, tearfulness, irritability, absenteeism, alcohol misuse or der-eliction of duty may be the presenting features of a personality disorder. Conflicts between people do not necessarily imply personality difficulties in the individuals concerned, but recurring interpersonal difficulties, with different people in various parts of an organisation, do suggest enduring problems in relationships which the individual brings to every new setting.

In organisations arranged more or less hierarchically, problems between boss and subordinate represent one common pattern. It is important to remember that any personality problems may be in the boss rather than the subordinate. There are increasing numbers of matrix organisations, where individuals report to three or more people, not always even in the same country, and many businesses are developing flat structures in which teamwork with peer groups is crucial. Both types of organisation can cause difficulties for people with personality disorders and make recognition of problems more tricky. Dysfunctional groups can have a damaging impact on a business and the ripple effect from one person with a personality disorder can be substantially greater than in a hierarchical organisation.

Problematic patterns of behaviour in the workplace

Six patterns of behaviour are particularly important in a work setting.

Obsessionality

Severely obsessional people are conscientious, careful, reliable and likely to attend scrupulously to detail and to check their work with extreme care. They may have difficulty dealing with workloads because of the time which care and checking take. Not infrequently, obsessional individuals are promoted to a decision-making position because of their reliability and the high quality of their work. Breakdown may then occur as a high level of rapid independent decision-making capacity does not usually accompany a marked degree of obsessionality.

Emotionality

Normally, sad events make people sad, uncertainties make people anxious and frustrations lead to irritability or anger. People with personality disorders may have difficulties with emotional experience and expressiveness: emotional responses may be of greater amplitude than is usual or appropriate; or mood swings may occur both upwards and downwards without any obvious preceding event. Unnatural cheerfulness, overactivity, unrealistic planning and depressed mood can all interfere with work performance and attendance.

Paranoid and schizoid tendencies

A sense of exploitation and mistrust in people with a paranoid tendency, and the cold, distant demeanour of people with a schizoid tendency, make the building of working relationships particularly difficult and this can have serious effects on teamwork, particularly if an organisation moves from a more formal 'vertical' structure to one based on informality and peer groups.

Aggressivity and irresponsibility

Impulsiveness, relative lack of concern for others, alcohol and drug misuse, and a tendency to aggression and rule violation make people with these personality disorders very disruptive in a work setting and positively dangerous in environments where safety is crucial.

Anxiousness

Preoccupation with physical symptoms can detract from work efficiency, and anxiety inappropriately attached to a stimulus like a phobia of underground, rail or air travel can make working arrangements complicated, particularly if an organisation expands to include distant or overseas locations.

Partnerships

People who meet at work not infrequently become partners. In situations where agreed rules (usually covert) about sexual relationships are broken, it is not unusual for one participant in the activity to have a personality problem. The clue is the repetition of the problematic activity in more than one setting; personality disorder not infrequently involves difficulty in restraining sexual impulses.

Summary

Personality difficulties predispose people to the experience of emotional distress or to problematic behaviour, sometimes in response to pressure, in particular in response to organisational and managerial actions which create difficulties for the individual. Whenever emotional or behavioural problems arise in relation to work, assessment of the situation should include the personalities involved, the organisational structure and any process of change within the working environment.

Potential employees bring inherent personality difficulties with them to an employer and prevention of personality problems in the workplace really means limiting their impact. It is therefore essential that the selection process involves an honest and comprehensive description of the job offered, to enable recruits to make sensible choices about what work they take on. In settings where a group of people work together, all members should ideally have a voice in the selection process, as obvious mismatches can spell disaster. Selectors should also ask realistic questions of referees and bear in mind previous absence records.

Once people are at work, changing work patterns should be addressed proactively. All individuals need appropriate training to give them both the competence and the confidence to adapt to changed job expectations. Line managers and human resource professionals should be alert for group or individual dysfunction at any time of major change in an organisation. The early involvement of occupational health staff, and job modifications if possible, may prevent a crisis. Seamless assimilation of occupational health units into the mainstream of business and organisational activities greatly enhances their efficacy. Access to occupational psychiatrists makes accurate diagnosis more likely than when all the organisational ills are attributed generally to 'stress'.

For those people whose 'breakdown' is recognised late, access to trained counsellors or employee assistance programmes may be enough to support their rehabilitation. In these circumstances it is essential that these professionals, with the employee's consent, give adequate feedback to the organisation so that potentially damaging situations can be addressed early. In other cases, cognitive–behavioural therapy with a suitably trained occupational health nurse or psychologist may be needed.

When every remedial process fails, in order to protect other members of the organisation, sympathetic termination of employment may be the only answer.

Reference

World Health Organization (1992) *Tenth Revision of the International Classification of Diseases* (ICD–10). Geneva: WHO.

CHAPTER 21

The role of mental health professionals

Steve McKeown and Susan Robson

Getting the best from mental health professionals

The aim of this chapter is to provide occupational health physicians with clear information about the roles, qualifications and competencies of the various mental health professions, so that they can make the most appropriate use of the advice and help available. The mental health team now includes psychiatrists, psychologists, cognitive–behavioural therapists, psychotherapists, counsellors and community psychiatric nurses.

Background

It helps to understand the context in which mental health services have developed – focused as they are around the *treatment* of mental illness. Occupational physicians enjoy a unique perspective on mental health which extends far beyond this. Occupational health intervention in the workplace includes *prevention, diagnosis, referral* and *liaison* with general practitioners and specialists and, by working with management, *rehabilitation*.

The problems are particularly acute in the National Health Service (NHS), where mental health service provision has declined in real terms over the past 20 years. As an inevitable consequence, NHS services are thinly spread, overloaded and overflowing with severely mentally ill patients, most suffering from a psychotic illness. The vast majority of these patients are unemployed. In some areas psychiatric services have virtually no resources available for patients other than the acutely disturbed. It is, therefore, extremely difficult for an occupational physician or general practitioner to organise an effective and speedy treatment package for someone who is moderately depressed, is suffering from occupational stress or has an early-stage alcohol problem.

Hence there has developed an industry devoted to providing assistance for mental health problems, as opposed to major mental illness. The positive face of this initiative is seen in innovative, effective treatment packages provided by properly trained, qualified and regulated mental health professionals. The down side is seen in the advertisements to be found in the classified sections of most local newspapers and magazines. An army of dubiously trained, underqualified and unsupervised therapists advertise a wide variety of services not subject to proper accreditation or quality control; some impressive-sounding qualifications can be bought on a franchise basis.

Equally inevitable has been the growth of a 'grey' area between the worlds of the respectable and the clearly disreputable. Some thorough research over the past five years has demonstrated what, with hindsight, may have been obvious: employee assistance programmes (EAPs) are only as good as the counsellors who provide them, quirky new treatments usually do not work, and there are no more valid quick fixes to be found in mental health treatment than in immunology or oncology. Occupational physicians remain guardians of science-based knowledge at a time when parapsychology and mythology are fashionable.

Mental health problems still carry a stigma which physical illness does not. In 2001, the Royal College of Psychiatrists launched a major campaign entitled 'Changing Minds' (http://www.stigma.org). This five-year campaign aims to increase public and professional under-standing of different mental health problems; to reduce the stigma of, and discrimination against, people suffering from these problems; and to close the gap between the different beliefs of health care professionals and the public about useful treatments and interventions. The problem which arises is where to draw the line. The traditional medical model of the patient as a passive victim of illness is increasingly irrelevant. Most mental health problems are not best treated by the application of a treatment from a well-meaning professional, whether that treatment consists of tablets, cranial osteopathy, analytical psychotherapy or any other intervention shrouded in mystique. With very few exceptions, mental health problems (in contrast to the psychoses) can be sensibly understood as problems or breakdowns in the life management skills or coping resources of the sufferer. Long-term solutions cannot, therefore, be achieved unless patients, as well as those around them, have a clear understanding of what has happened, and accurate and accessible information about the problem and its significance, so that they can be equipped with the relevant skills to overcome the difficulty. Physical treatments, such as medication, may sometimes be part of this process. It will be obvious from the above that most problems require a well-orchestrated team of professionals, communicating openly and regularly with each other. The remainder of this chapter is intended to assist a clear understanding of the role of each profession.

Psychiatrists

Psychiatrists are medically qualified doctors specialising in the diagnosis and treatment of mental illness; some of their main tasks are identification, classification and diagnosis, and a generation ago their perspective was limited to diagnostic assessments and the prescription of treatments. A minority of psychiatrists in the UK were trained as psychotherapists, but psychotherapy treatments such as psychoanalysis never flourished there as they did in mainland Europe and North America.

Senior psychiatrists are recognised under the Mental Health Act, which is designed as a mechanism for ensuring that patients who pose a danger to themselves or others can be hospitalised and treated without their consent. In many areas services are sectorised and organised geographically. The role of most psychiatrists has metamorphosed into that of team leader for a mental health team of professionals (members of which are described below). There has also been increasing overlap with clinical psychologists as psychological treatments have gained in prominence. Psychiatrists retain specialist skill in the clinical assessment and diagnosis of patients, and the demand for this function from lawyers, insurance companies and employers is ever growing.

Psychologists

After completing their first degree, psychologists undertake postgraduate training (often up to doctorate level) in clinical, occupational, educational or child psychology.

Clinical psychologists have a well-established place in the mental health team. Their main task used to be measurement and assessment through the design and development of psychometric tests, and operationally defining behaviour and personality problems in ways that can be measured. Psychologists, particularly in the USA, spearheaded cognitive–behavioural therapy (CBT), in the 1970s, both as a reaction against long-winded and intangible forms of psychotherapy and as a means of providing quicker, cheaper and more measurable treatments. There is now considerable overlap between clinical psychologists and psychiatrists.

Clinical psychologists within the NHS work usually from clinical psychology departments, in which waiting lists of more than nine months for assessment and treatment are common. To reduce this bottleneck, psychologists increasingly undertake sessions in primary care centres, following the initiative of the psychiatric outreach clinic.

Cognitive–behavioural therapists

Cognitive–behavioural therapy promotes detailed understanding and modification of the thinking processes and behaviours that cause anxiety problems and perpetuate depression. The best cognitive–behavioural therapists start with a professional grounding in psychiatric nursing, occupational therapy or are psychiatrists or psychologists who specialise in CBT. Treatment consists of a programme of sessions (usually 6 to 15) interspersed with homework assignments. Hence adequate motivation from the patient is essential. Good CBT is well organised, transparent and progresses towards specified goals quantified regularly by the therapist and patient. Research studies repeatedly demonstrate that CBT combined with physical treatments is strikingly more effective than either treatment in isolation for depression and anxiety.

Psychotherapists, counsellors, EAP providers and others

As described above, the increasing demand for mental health treatments has led to numerous misconceptions, some of which have taken surprisingly strong root. Among these are the following irrational beliefs:

- longer treatments are more effective than shorter treatments
- a single counsellor can handle any problem, from sexual abuse to bereavement
- exposure to a traumatic incident automatically requires an immediate course of counselling
- counselling as part of an employee assistance programme (EAP) improves mental health
- anybody can identify clinical depression
- a therapist or counsellor can function separately, in complete confidence, from the rest of the treatment team.

Solid evidence now exists that all these assumptions are incorrect.

Every doctor and psychologist will have had the benefit of a formal scientific training, which is too useful to be casually abandoned. This does not justify intellectual arrogance, but it should signal caution in the face of unlikely, untested or counterintuitive treatments which have not undergone rigorous scrutiny.

Community psychiatric nurses

In theory, community psychiatric nurses (CPNs) are the primary contacts of the community mental health team; they able to supervise and support those with mental illness, as well as to provide anxiety management training and CBT. In reality many are so overwhelmed by demand that they have little time except for the severely ill. A significant number have acquired extra skills in CBT in order to move to a role where they deliver out-patient or day-patient treatment.

De facto members of the mental health service

Finally, there are three other agencies who are de facto members of the mental health service and whose input needs to be recognised, integrated and respected.

First, and obvious from the above, there is a considerable and increasing need for acquisition of better self-management skills to maintain and improve mental health. As well as anxiety and panic management skills and rational thinking, mental health requires effective assertiveness, time management and communication skills. Increasingly there are productive liaisons between mental health professionals and human resource, organisational development and personnel professionals.

Second, occupational physicians and general practitioners are a vital part of a comprehensive team. As well as their involvement at the stage of problem identification, diagnosis and referral, active management of sickness absence, rehabilitation back into work, identification of work-related stress issues and maintenance of a healthy organisational culture depend on active involvement at this level.

Third, it is obvious that the patient must be regarded not as a passive recipient of treatment, but as an autonomous and educable partner in the process of achieving and maintaining health. Motivation, enthusiasm and active investment in the formation of a strong therapeutic alliance is the ideal, and it is unlikely that any problem will be satisfactorily resolved without shared ownership by the sufferer.

Mental health professionals and occupational health

While many severely mentally ill patients may well be temporarily unemployable, they do qualify as disabled under the Disability Discrimination Act and there are those who, with successful treatment, may well seek to return to or remain in employment. As a result, it is essential that the various professionals (mental health, occupational health and management) work closely and, where appropriate, advise and provide reasonable adjustment and support to enable a person's occupational rehabilitation.

The nature of the most commonly cited work-related medical conditions is changing from those seen at the beginning of the 20th century, such as occupational lung diseases, to musculoskeletal and increasingly stress- and anxiety-related problems. This is especially true of those professions, such as teaching, medicine and the police, where there is a duty of care towards others and where psychiatric and psychological conditions now account for the majority of ill health retirement and sickness absence. More than ever before, occupational physicians are looking to mental health professionals to provide practical, professional and specialist advice.

Future trends

The pace of change in mental health seems likely to accelerate. Expectations continue to grow but resources are more limited. Two more fundamental developments are proving to be useful.

The first is preventive maintenance. Individual life management skills portfolios can be assessed before problems arise and the necessary skills training implemented proactively.

The second development is the harnessing of the power of information technology. Interactive packages allow computers to undertake screening, assessment and skills development programmes which are reliable and consistent. These can supplement traditional, face-to-face interviews.

CHAPTER 22

The role of the liaison psychiatrist

Andrew Hodgkiss and David Snashall

What is liaison psychiatry?

Liaison psychiatry is a growing sub-speciality of general adult psychiatry. There are about 60 consultant liaison psychiatrists in Britain and 30 specialist registrars in training. Liaison psychiatry seeks to address the mental health needs of patients in the setting of the general hospital. This includes attenders at the accident and emergency (A & E) department as well as in-patients and out-patients under the care of physicians, surgeons and obstetricians. In addition to patients presenting to the hospital with deliberate self-harm or obvious severe mental illness, liaison psychiatry involves the treatment of patients with comorbidity of physical and psychiatric illness and with somatoform disorders. Liaison psychiatry arguably includes super-specialities, such as perinatal psychiatry, psychosocial oncology, psychosexual medicine, neuropsychiatry and eating disorders. Despite the fact that there are specialist psychiatrists in substance misuse, drug and alcohol problems can constitute a significant part of the liaison psychiatrist's workload.

Liaison psychiatrists differ from general adult psychiatrists leading community mental health teams in several important respects. Liaison psychiatrists see general hospital patients regardless of their home address, are based in the general hospital, tend to have very few psychiatric beds and have special experience with non-psychotic patients. Many also have expertise in psychological treatments such as cognitive–behavioural therapy (CBT). Most liaison psychiatrists will accept appropriate referrals (people under 65 years of age) from local general practitioners and occupational health physicians. It is psychogeriatricians who usually offer a liaison service to their local geriatricians.

Who should be referred to a liaison psychiatrist?

Mood disturbance in chronic physical illness

It is now well established that the prevalence of mood disturbance among people with a physical illness is high, but detecting it is not easy. First, it is tempting to assume that psychological illness is an inevitable consequence of, for example, a diagnosis of cancer or multiple sclerosis. This is not true. Second, the clinician cannot rely on biological symptoms (such as early morning waking, weight loss and the loss of libido) to diagnose depression in people who have a chronic physical illness, because pain, cachexia or nausea due to the medical condition and its treatment may cause such symptoms. Instead, the psychological and behavioural symptoms of depression must be sought. These include hopelessness, helplessness, worthlessness, guilt, hypo-chondriacal preoccupations, suicidal ideas and plans, loss of interest, self-neglect, social withdrawal, indecision and poor concentration. Some medical conditions obscure the signs of depression; for example, the mask-like face and bradykinesia of Parkinson's disease can disguise mental state signs such as psychomotor retardation.

The vigorous treatment of mood disturbance, once detected, in patients with chronic medical conditions is worthwhile and rewarding. It can make an enormous difference to their quality of life. It can improve compliance with medical treatment. And it can influence the prognosis of the medical condition.

The safest choice of antidepressant in various medical conditions is one area where the liaison psychiatrist has expertise. Some patients, while acknowledging that they are depressed, refuse antidepressant medication because they cannot face taking more tablets. In such cases liaison psychiatrists can offer cognitive therapy, which is as effective as antidepressants for mild to moderate depressive illness.

Somatoform disorders

'Somatisation' is a highly fashionable term but there is often confusion about its meaning. Some use it to refer to any somatic symptom that cannot be explained by a medical diagnosis. Others take it to mean that some sort of psychological distress lies behind the somatic symptoms. The latter is the more common usage and includes an aetiological statement that is indebted to Freud's notion of 'conversion' from the psychological realm to the physical. Somatisation is a process and there is a wide spectrum of severity. Somatised symptoms can last minutes ('that man's giving me a headache') or years. Acute somatisation accounts for a substantial proportion of consultations with general practitioners. Most of these illnesses are self-limiting. It is the smaller number of chronic somatisers who require the attention of a liaison psychiatrist.

The psychiatric classification of these chronic somatoform disorders changes every few years. For practical purposes they can be grouped under four headings.

Conversion disorder

This is closest to classical Freudian hysteria and is much more common in women than in men. The onset is in early adulthood. The somatic symptom is not consciously produced. The clinician finds the symptom to be loaded with meaning in relation to the patient's autobiography or psychological conflicts. Examples include pseudo-seizures, mono-plegias, aphonia and bizarre gait. Treatment may include behavioural approaches, abreaction or analytical psychotherapy.

Pain disorder

Pain without lesion is separated from conversion symptoms because it often reflects depressive illness rather than being symbolic of anything. Unexplained chronic pain in the low back, face, arm or pelvis is very common. The clinical picture often becomes complicated by analgesic dependence. Treatment includes low-dose tricyclic antidepressants and cognitive–behavioural pain management strategies.

Somatisation disorder

This is the most extreme end of the spectrum. These patients have multiple somatic symptoms in several body systems and use huge amounts of health service resources. They have multiple investigations and surgical interventions. Some studies have identified such patients by simply weighing hospital notes. Treatment is aimed at containing the grossly abnormal illness behaviour through regular contact with one trusted doctor who listens and examines but declines to refer on or investigate each new complaint.

Hypochondriasis

Hypochondriasis is a disorder of belief – these patients are troubled by the belief that they are seriously physically ill and they cannot be reassured to the contrary. It can vary from an understandable preoccupy-ing idea (overvalued idea) to an unshakeable certainty (hypochondriacal delusion). The commonest cause of hypochondriasis is depressive illness. The difference between a patient with conversion disorder and a hypochondriacal patient is considerable. In a conversion disorder the somatic symptom simply occurs and the patient often has remarkably little concern as to its seriousness (*belle indifference*), while in hypo-chondriasis there may be few somatic symptoms at all but intense concern about the possibility of life-threatening disease.

In the work setting, hypochondriasis has to be distinguished from frank malingering. Management includes treatment for depression and CBT (which includes the banning of reassurance).

Chronic fatigue

This rather mixed group of patients, some lacking energy because of depressive illness, some with persistent post-viral fatigue, some with unexplained fatigue, should be referred for assessment if fatigue has lasted six months or more. Treatments include CBT, graded exercise and the judicious use of non-sedative antidepressants. (See Chapter 17 for a more detailed discussion of chronic fatigue.)

Recurrent deliberate self-harm

Assessing patients who have deliberately harmed themselves – including those who repeatedly mutilate themselves ('cutters'), those who have poisoned themselves and those who have made more violent suicide attempts – is a large part of the liaison psychiatry workload in the general hospital. For example, 1000 cases of deliberate self-harm present to the A&E department of St Thomas' Hospital, London, each year. Those identified as having obvious psychiatric disorders are referred to a community mental health team or psychiatric ward. But a small proportion repeatedly self-harm in the absence of obvious psychiatric disorder. This group can be highly problematic and time-consuming. Some liaison psychiatrists offer psychological treatment for such patients.

Perinatal psychiatric problems

Liaison psychiatrists are keen to see pregnant women with histories of schizophrenia, unipolar or bipolar affective disorder, puerperal psychosis, or severe postnatal depression to help plan for the birth. They tend to have links with mother-and-baby units and can facilitate planned or emergency admission. They also have expertise in the management of postnatal depression, especially the vexed question of prescribing antidepressants to breastfeeding mothers.

Psychosexual problems

Most liaison psychiatrists have an interest in psychosexual problems, particularly those of people who have a chronic physical illness.

Eating disorders

Anorexia nervosa and bulimia nervosa should be referred to liaison psychiatry unless the local community mental health team has experience in such work or specialist eating disorder services exist.

The occupational physician, when seeking a specialist report on patients with these groups of disorders, should consider approaching a liaison psychiatrist.

Further reading

Bass, C. (ed.) (1990) *Somatisation: Physical Symptoms and Psychological Illness*. Oxford: Blackwell Scientific.

Guthrie, E. & Creed, F. (eds) (1996) *Seminars in Liaison Psychiatry*. London: Gaskell.

Halligan, P. W., Bass, C. & Marshall, J. C. (eds) (2001) *Contemporary Approaches to the Study of Hysteria*. Oxford: Oxford Medical Publications.

Ramirez, A. & House, A. (1997) ABC of mental health. Common mental health problems in hospital. *British Medical Journal*, **314**, 1679–1681.

Index

Abbreviated Mental Test Score 142
absenteeism
    costs 29–32
    incidence 35
    policies 43–44
Access to Health Records Act (1990) 17
Access to Medical Reports Act (1988) 17
aggression 146
agnosia 140
agoraphobia 85, 115
alcohol misuse 98–104
    and depression 89
    policies 43–44, 102–103
Alexander & Bridge (consultants) 7–8
Alzheimer's disease 138, 140
anorexia nervosa 109–113, 157–158
antidepressants 87, 92–93, 155, 156
antipsychotic drugs 135–136
anxiety 78–80, 82–87
    in chronic physical illness 155
    personality disorder 146
    travel phobia 85–86, 114–120
    treatment 86–87
apraxia 140
Assessment of Motor and Process Skills
    (AMPS) 143
AstraZeneca 53–59
attention 138

Banham, J. 30
Barclays Bank 31
Beck, A.T. 90–91
Beck Anxiety Inventory 91
Beck Depression Inventory 90
benzodiazepines 87
bereavement 89–90
beta-blockers 87

bipolar affective disorder (manic-
    depressive illness) 78–80, 118
brain tumours 139, 140
Briner, R.B. 37
bulimia nervosa 109–113, 157–158
bullying 96
business case 28–33

CALM programme 55–58
change
    employees' attitudes 3–4
    management 1–9, 43
    organisational culture 4–6, 43
    as psychosocial hazard 40
    RATIO programme 4–8
    relocation 5
    reorganisation 6–8
    success factors 8–9
    support programmes 2–8
chronic fatigue syndrome 20, 127–131
chronic physical illness 155
claustrophobia 115
Clothier Report (1991) 109, 111
cognitive–behavioural therapy 86, 116–
    117, 131, 150–151, 154
cognitive therapy 91–92, 155
communications 38–39, 43
community psychiatric nurses (CPNs) 151
compartmentalisation 70–71
concentration 138
confidentiality 16–17, 76–77
Conner, D.R. 68
conversion disorder 156
Cooper, C.L. 51, 57
counselling 149, 151
    appropriate 81
    CALM programme 55–58

Counselling and Life Management (CALM) programme 55–58
Covey, S.R. 69
Cox, T. 37
crèches 44
Creutzfeld–Jacob disease 143
critical incidents 121–126

Data Protection Act (1998) 12, 17–18
delirium 78–80, 138
delusional disorders 132–137
dementia 78–80, 138, 140
depression 78–80, 88–93
    in chronic physical illness 155
Disability Discrimination Act (1995) 10, 11, 20–21, 36, 42, 131, 136, 152
dismissal, unfair 19
Doherty, N. 32
dothiepin 87
drug misuse 105–108
dysthymia 90

e-mail 39
eating disorders 109–113, 157–158
emotionality 145–146
employee assistance programmes (EAPs) 149, 151
Employment Relations Act (1999) 19
Employment Rights Act (1996) 11
energy, enhancing 70
eye movement desensitisation and reprocessing (EMDR) 125–126

Farnsworth case 10
Farrell, M. 105
fatigue 139
    chronic 157
    chronic fatigue syndrome 20, 127–131
fear of flying 114–117
Fisher, A.G. 143
Fit For Work programme 23–27
flexitime 44
Folstein, M.S. 142
frontal lobe syndromes 139–140
functional disorders 140–141

Gandhi, Mahatma 71
General Health Questionnaire (GHQ) 57
General Medical Council (GMC) 16–17
general stress model 37
generalised anxiety disorder 82–3
Glaxo Pharmaceuticals UK (GPUK) 1–9
Goldberg, D. 57
Gratton, K. 7

hallucinations 132–133
harassment, policies 43–44
head injury 139, 140
health education programmes 31–32
health promotion packages 44
Health and Safety Executive (HSE)
    guidance on pre-employment health screening 11
    guidance on stress at work 12–13
Health and Safety at Work etc. Act (1974) 12, 36, 108
Heron, R.J.L. 57
Hospital Anxiety and Depression Scale 91
human resources, statistics 41–42
Human Rights Act (1998) 18
hypochondriasis 156–157

interpersonal relationships 41
irresponsibility 146

jet lag 118–119
job specifications 41
Jones, G. 16
Jones, N. 28

Kapadia case 21
Kim, W.C. 7
Korsakov's syndrome 139
Lance, Sean 4–5
Leading Edge Forum Ltd 7
legal aspects 10–21
liaison psychiatry 154–155
life balance 69–70
lifestyle 68–74
Lishman, W.A. 138
litigation costs 29–30
lofepramine 93
London Electricity case 23–27
Lowndes, S.N. 28

Management of Health and Safety at Work Regulations (1999) 13, 36, 108, 123
manic–depressive illness 78–80, 118
Marks & Spencer 60–67
Markus, A. 90
Mauborgue, R. 7
mefloquine 117–118
Meltzer, H. 58
memory 139
mental health (mental well-being)
    and business success 58
    models 53–54
    resilience 68
Mental Health Act (1983) 18–19, 150

mental health policies
  business case 28–33
  developing 34–46
  employee surveys 57–58
  evaluation 57–58
  guidelines 54–55
  safety, health and environment (SHE) 54–55
  team approach 53–59
mental health problems
  assessment 75–81, 111–113
  costs 23–24, 29–32
  diagnosis 78–80
  emergency treatment in the workplace 18–19
  employee support 45
  foreseeability 14
  general stress model 37
  legal aspects 10–21
  management *see* mental health policies
  occupational health interventions 96–97
  physical hazard model 37
  pre-employment assessment 11–12
  preventing 12–16, 23–27, 31–32, 43–45
  psychosocial hazards 38–41
  and recruitment 10–12, 111–113
  referrals 80–81
  rehabilitation *see* rehabilitation
  risk *see* risk
  stigma 149
mental health professionals 148–153
mental state examination 78, 142
Miller, D.M. 35
Mini-Mental State Examination (MMSE) 142
Misrepresentation Act (1976) 12
Misuse of Drugs Act (1971) 108
morale 39
Morgan, J.H. 111
Morgan case 20–21
Muir, J. 29
multiple sclerosis 139, 140
Murray Parkes, C. 90
myalgic encephalomyelitis 127–131

National Health Service (NHS) changes 3, 4, 6
neurasthenia 127–131
neurotic symptoms 138
noise 51, 52

O'Brien case 11
obsessional–compulsive disorder (OCD) 87–88

obsessionality 145
Occupational Stress Indicator (OSI) 57, 61
occupational toxins 77, 138, 139, 140, 142
organic disorders 138–143
organisational capability 73–74
organisational change *see* change
organisational culture 4–6, 38
organisational styles 38–40

pain disorder 156
panic disorder 84–85, 115
paranoid tendency 146
parietal lobe symptoms 140
Parkinson's disease 139
perinatal disorders 157
person–environment fit 44
personal injury claims 13, 30
personality disorder 78–80, 109, 144–147
personnel policies, inadequate 40
phobic anxiety 85–86
physical hazard model 37, 45–46
physical illness, chronic 155
poisoning 77, 138, 139, 140, 142
Post Office 32
post-traumatic stress disorder 121–126
  absences 32
post-viral fatigue syndrome (PVFS) 127–131
pressure
  see also stress
  management 60–67, 71–73
  versus stress 47
Pressure Management Indicator 51, 61–67
psychiatric assessment interviews 75–81
psychiatric disorders *see* mental health problems
psychiatrists 150
psychologists 150
psychosexual disorders 157
psychosocial hazards 38–41
psychotherapy 151

RATIO programme 4–8
Rayner, C. 96
recruitment
  and mental health problems 10–12, 111–113
  schizophrenia 137
Rees, L. 141
referrals 80–81
rehabilitation 44
  drug misuse 107–108
  schizophrenia 135–136

relocation 5
resilience 68, 72–73
risk
    assessment 36–37, 41–42, 78
    management 23–27, 96–97
    reduction 42–45
role conflict 41
Role Interventional Assessment Tool
    (RIAT) 26–27

Saunders, B. 107
schizoid tendency 146
schizophrenia 78–80, 118, 132–137
SCOFF questionnaire 111–112
selective serotonin reuptake inhibitors
    (SSRIs) 87, 92–93
self-harm 93–96, 157
Seligman, M. 68
sexual relationships 146
Smith, A. 35
Snaith, R.P. 91
social phobias 86
somatisation disorder 82, 156
somatoform disorders 155–157
stigma 149
Strang, J. 105
stress
    see also pressure
    audit 42
    clinical presentations 49–50
    definitions 47
    effect on work 50
    interventions 50–52
    job-specific factors 40–41
    and management skills 40, 43
    measurement 61–62
    organisational factors 38–40
    post-traumatic see post-traumatic stress
        disorder
    pre-employment assessment 42
    v. pressure 47
    prevention 12–13
    prognosis 50
    risk assessment 24–27, 41–42
    training workshops 54–55, 57, 58,
        64–65
    women 44, 64

stress management 51–52
    pressure management 60–67, 71–73
    training programmes 44, 65–67
stress-related illness
    absenteeism 29–32
    assessment 77–78
    causes 48
    costs 29–32
    incidence 34–36
    interventions 31–32
    legal aspects 10–21
substance misuse 78–80
    alcohol see alcohol misuse
    drug misuse 105–108
    policies 43–44
suicide 93–96
syphilis 140

Taylor, R. 29
temporal lobe symptoms 140
Thackrah, C.T. 60
thought disorder 132–133
thyroid dysfunction 139, 142
traits 144
travel phobia 85–86, 114–120
Tyson, S. 32

unfair dismissal 19

vascular lesions 140
venlafaxine 92, 93
violence at work 121–126
    policies 43–44

Walker case 13, 30, 36, 44
Welch, J. 30, 31
Wellcome UK 8
Williams, S. 51, 71
women 44, 64
work overload 41
working hours
    policies 44
    and social life 41
Working Time Regulations (1998) 15–16

Zantac (ranitidine) 8
Zigmond, A.S. 91